AF807138

Mechanical Ventilation in Critical Care Transport

Susan R. Wilcox • Jason Cohen
Michael Frakes
Editors

Mechanical Ventilation in Critical Care Transport

Springer

Editors
Susan R. Wilcox
Boston MedFlight
Bedford, MA, USA

Jason Cohen
Boston MedFlight
Bedford, MA, USA

Michael Frakes
Boston MedFlight
Bedford, MA, USA

ISBN 978-3-031-66781-7 ISBN 978-3-031-66782-4 (eBook)
https://doi.org/10.1007/978-3-031-66782-4

© The Editor(s) (if applicable) and The Author(s), under exclusive license to Springer Nature Switzerland AG 2024
This work is subject to copyright. All rights are solely and exclusively licensed by the Publisher, whether the whole or part of the material is concerned, specifically the rights of translation, reprinting, reuse of illustrations, recitation, broadcasting, reproduction on microfilms or in any other physical way, and transmission or information storage and retrieval, electronic adaptation, computer software, or by similar or dissimilar methodology now known or hereafter developed.
The use of general descriptive names, registered names, trademarks, service marks, etc. in this publication does not imply, even in the absence of a specific statement, that such names are exempt from the relevant protective laws and regulations and therefore free for general use.
The publisher, the authors and the editors are safe to assume that the advice and information in this book are believed to be true and accurate at the date of publication. Neither the publisher nor the authors or the editors give a warranty, expressed or implied, with respect to the material contained herein or for any errors or omissions that may have been made. The publisher remains neutral with regard to jurisdictional claims in published maps and institutional affiliations.

This Springer imprint is published by the registered company Springer Nature Switzerland AG
The registered company address is: Gewerbestrasse 11, 6330 Cham, Switzerland

If disposing of this product, please recycle the paper.

For Suzanne K. Wedel, MD

Acknowledgments

The authors would like to thank Evie Marcolini, MD, and Ani Aydin, MD. They are tireless advocates for critical care transport and mechanical ventilation education, and their collaboration on a prior mechanical ventilation textbook inspired this work.

We would also like to thank the Boston MedFlight clinicians. Our colleagues are thoughtful, knowledgeable, and dedicated, and they inspire us with their constant enthusiasm for education.

Lastly, we thank our patients. It is an honor and a privilege to be trusted to care for critically ill and injured patients in transport across New England.

Contents

Introduction

1

Susan R. Wilcox, Michael Frakes, and Jason Cohen

Mechanical ventilation is one of the most common procedures in all critical care, including critical care transport. Yet, despite the frequency with which patients are intubated and ventilated, the management of ventilation poses significant risks to the patient. Whether patients are intubated for acute hypoxemic or hypercapnic respiratory failure, trauma, intracranial hemorrhages, or their overall clinical course, the need for artificial ventilation is a marker of significant illness. As clinicians frequently care for ventilated critically ill patients, clinicians can become numb to the significance of mechanical ventilation. However, initiating and maintaining mechanical ventilation requires great vigilance, as these patients have high rates of adverse events, especially in transport.

Historically, mechanical ventilation has been a peripheral part of paramedic, nurse, and emergency physician practices, with many of the details of ventilation left to Intensivists and Respiratory Therapists. However, in the transport environment, understanding the nuances of mechanical ventilation and its impact on physiology is extremely important. Respiratory therapists and critical care physicians are essential critical care team members, but they may not be available in austere or remote locations, and consultation may not always be practical. While the transport world mandates substantial clinician autonomy, the data supporting the importance of good ventilator management in all critically ill patients continues to increase. This means that more than ever, transport clinicians are responsible for managing ventilators according to evidence-based principles.

This text focuses on managing mechanical ventilation and its impact on physiology, focusing on the transport environment. While other texts focus on ICU ventilation management, we recognize that the transport environment is unique. In contrast to other transport-specific books, this text highlights the clinical context for all

S. R. Wilcox (✉) · M. Frakes · J. Cohen
Boston MedFlight, Bedford, MA, USA
e-mail: susan.r.wilcox@lahey.org

© The Author(s), under exclusive license to Springer Nature Switzerland AG 2024

S. R. Wilcox et al. (eds.), *Mechanical Ventilation in Critical Care Transport*,
https://doi.org/10.1007/978-3-031-66782-4_1

patients, emphasizing special patient populations, including neonates and pediatric patients.

A few words about the style and function of these educational materials are in order. The editors assume readers are knowledgeable and experienced in transport medicine but seek mechanical ventilation education. As such, significant details of other medical management are beyond the scope of this text. To develop the concepts around ventilation, many examples and illustrations are set in the hospital, using detailed ICU ventilators as instructional instruments. However, the principles are specified for the out-of-hospital environment. Using some principles of adult learning theory, this text starts with basic definitions, deliberately uses spaced reiteration to provide the same ideas in different contexts, and emphasizes clinical scenarios. Hence, if the information seems repetitive, that is by design to enhance understanding and recall. We have included references to other chapters addressing the same information where appropriate.

The objectives of this text are to

1. Familiarize transport clinicians with common terms in mechanical ventilation
2. Review key principles of pulmonary physiology relevant to both mechanical ventilation and specific to transport
3. Understand the interpretation of blood gases as related to the management of the ventilated patient
4. Discuss the basic principles of selecting ventilator settings
5. Develop strategies for caring for ventilated patients with ARDS, asthma, COPD, trauma, and neurologic injury
6. Provide information specific to caring for ventilated neonates and pediatric patients
7. Assess and respond to emergencies during mechanical ventilation

Terminology and Definitions

2

Mark S. Saia

Physiology Terms

Understanding the principles of respiratory physiology is important to understanding mechanical ventilation.

Ventilation has two definitions. First, ventilation is the fluctuation of air in and out of the lungs or through a portion of the lungs (Sometimes, in the operating room, clinicians may use "one-lung ventilation," with one lung collapsed and the other receiving airflow.). Additionally, when describing physiologic principles, "ventilation" refers to just a portion of the lung. In the second definition, because the diffusion of carbon dioxide is so closely related to the amount of air moved, the removal of carbon dioxide is often referred to as "ventilation" as well.

Perfusion is the blood flow through the lungs or a portion of the lungs. Perfusion is a major determinant of oxygenation, as the more blood flow that occurs, the more oxygen is picked up by the hemoglobin.

V/Q ratio and **V/Q matching** are the terms used to describe the relationship between ventilation (V) and perfusion (Q). In a perfect system, the ratio would be 1. When the ventilation is high, but there is no perfusion (a ratio of ∞), this is dead space. When the ventilation is nil but the perfusion is high (a ratio of 0), this is a shunt. Even in healthy people, different portions of the lung will have variable V/Q ratios. In pathology, patients can have shunts, dead space, and every relationship in between.

Airway resistance refers to the impedance to airflow throughout the system during the respiratory cycle. Normal airway resistance is ≤ 5 cmH_2O, but even a large value endotracheal tube increases resistance from that value for non-intubated patients [1]. Examples of high resistance would be a patient with bronchospasm, airway inflammation, a small endotracheal tube, or increased mucus.

M. S. Saia (✉)
Boston MedFlight, Bedford, MA, USA
e-mail: Mark.Saia@bostonmedflight.org

© The Author(s), under exclusive license to Springer Nature Switzerland AG 2024

S. R. Wilcox et al. (eds.), *Mechanical Ventilation in Critical Care Transport*,
https://doi.org/10.1007/978-3-031-66782-4_2

Respiratory system compliance refers to the distensibility of the lungs and is impacted by the rest of the system, including the chest wall and the abdomen [2]. Compliance is the opposite of **elastance**, or the ability to snap back into place. Lungs with a low compliance or high elastic recoil tend to have difficulty with inhalation and are often referred to as "stiff" lungs [3]. A clinical example of poor compliance would be a patient with acute respiratory distress syndrome (ARDS) or a restrictive lung disease such as pulmonary fibrosis. In contrast, highly compliant lungs, or ones with a low elastic recoil, tend to have more difficulty in the exhalation process, as seen in obstructive lung diseases. Normal lung compliance is approximately 100 ml/cmH_2O.

Derecruitment is large-scale atelectasis, resulting in the loss of surface area for gas exchange and often a decrease in compliance. It is a common cause of hypoxemia in intubated patients. However, increasing positive end-expiratory pressure (PEEP) can minimize or even reverse it.

Recruitment is the application of sustained pressure to reopen collapsed or atelectatic areas of the lung [3, 4]. This pressure can be negative in a spontaneously breathing patient or positive in a ventilated patient.

Predicted body weight (PBW) is the expected physiologic weight of a patient, formulaically determined by the height and sex as defined at birth. PBW is a reflection of the volume of the lungs. The absolute body weight may impact other factors in ventilation, such as CO_2 production or the pressures needed to generate tidal volume, but it does not impact lung volumes. The PBW, therefore, determines the preferred tidal volume. The PBW formula for men is: PBW (kg) = 50 + 2.3 (height (in) – 60), while for women it is: PBW (kg) = 45.5 + 2.3 (height (in) – 60) [2]. Note that while similar to "ideal body weight" as is used for some medication dosing, this formula is different.

Shunt is a major cause of hypoxemia in ventilated patients. In the lung, it refers to an area with no (or ineffective) ventilation and preserved perfusion.

Dead space is another cause of hypoxemia and, if large enough, can lead to hypercapnia. It is an area of the lung that is being ventilated but not perfused.

Introduction to the Ventilator

Control or target variables are the parameters clinicians set on the ventilator [3, 4]. Depending upon the mode chosen, different variables may be selected. For example, the tidal volume would be the control variable in a volume-targeted mode.

Conditional variables, or **dependent variables** in mechanical ventilation, result from the selections of the clinicians [3, 4]. The tidal volume and respiratory rate are set parameters in volume-controlled modes, while the pressure is a conditional variable. In pressure-controlled modes, the pressure and respiratory rate are set, while

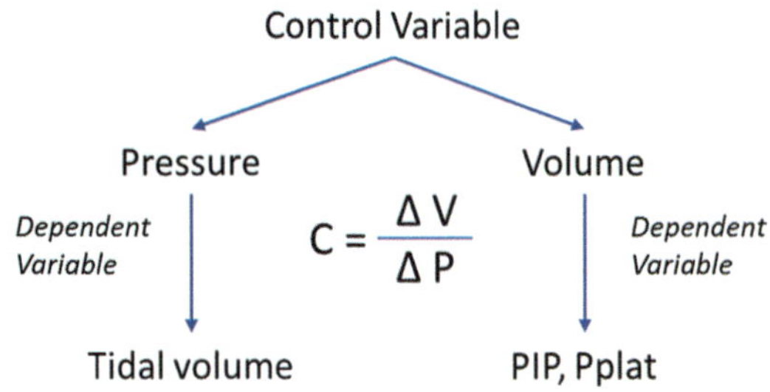

Fig. 2.1 Diagram of set or controlled variables, illustrating the dependent or conditional variables. Compliance, *C*, is the relationship between the change in volume divided by the change in pressure

the tidal volume is a conditional variable and can vary from breath to breath based on such variables, including resistance and compliance. Figure 2.1 shows this relationship.

Trigger is the set factor on a ventilator that initiates inspiration. Depending on the mode chosen, a breath can be pressure-triggered, flow-triggered, or time-triggered [3, 4].

Cycle refers to how the ventilator determines the end of inspiration and the beginning of exhalation. For example, a mechanical ventilator can be volume, pressure, or time-cycled [3, 4].

Phases of Mechanical Breathing

The initiation phase is the beginning of the breath. The breath can be triggered either by the patient (making a respiratory effort) or the ventilator (when it is time for another breath, given the settings entered by the clinician). With patient-initiated breaths, the waveforms show a slight negative deflection (negative pressure) in the pressure tracing, as shown in Fig. 2.2.

Note that this figure represents two respiratory cycles over approximately 4 s.

Inspiratory phase is the part of the respiratory cycle when air flows into the lungs, resulting in the desired pressure or tidal volume, as set by the clinician. The respiratory rate determines the duration of the inspiratory time (I-time), and the clinician sets I-time in pressure control or the clinician sets the flow rate in volume control. The inspiratory phase is shown in the diagram in Fig. 2.3. Note that this diagram shows one respiratory cycle but includes both pressure and flow waveforms.

Plateau phase is not a normal part of the respiratory cycle but is used for diagnostic purposes. When a patient is on volume-cycled ventilation, and the team wants to check the plateau pressure, which is the pressure distending the alveoli, they perform an inspiratory hold maneuver [2]. This results in the cessation of flow, illustrated in Fig. 2.4. The plateau is marked in red in the first respiratory cycle.

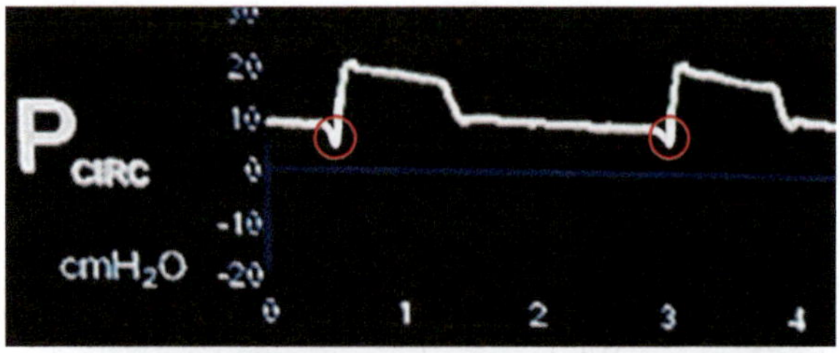

Fig. 2.2 Waveform illustrating initiation phase or triggering

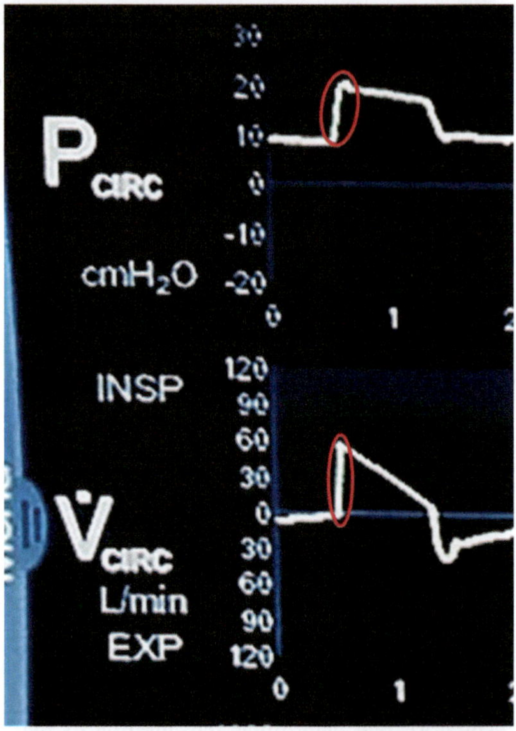

Fig. 2.3 Waveform illustrating inspiratory phase

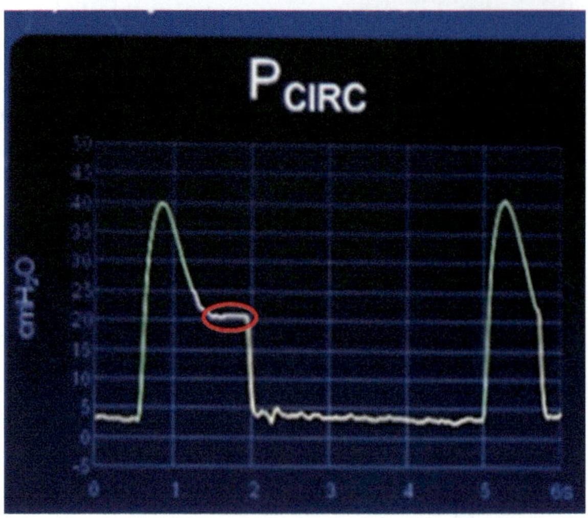

Fig. 2.4 Waveform illustrating plateau phase

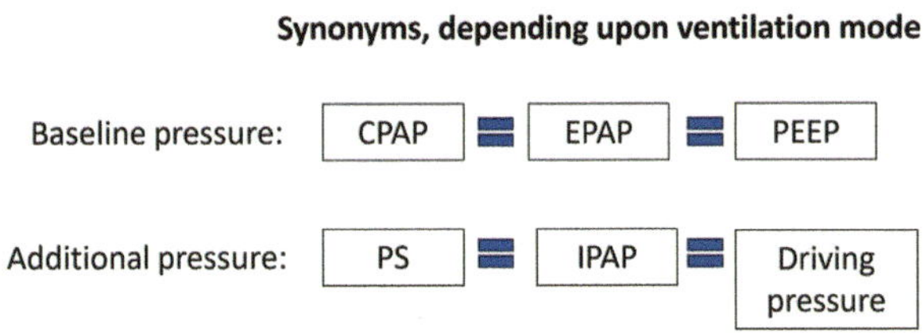

Fig. 6.6 Many terms have similar meanings, but by convention, are each used in different modes of ventilation. Understanding that the concepts behind the terms are the same helps with comprehension

Synchronized Intermittent Mandatory Ventilation

Synchronized intermittent mandatory ventilation (SIMV) combines assist control and pressure support ventilation modes. A mandatory minimum rate and breath type (with a set volume or pressure) is selected, and all patient-triggered breaths beyond this minimum get PSV support. This backup degree of support is set much the same way as AC mode. The clinician predetermines either a tidal volume or driving pressure, a FiO_2, and a minimum number of breaths per minute. This will be delivered even if the patient becomes apneic. If the patient starts to breathe more than this minimum rate, then each patient-triggered breath will receive an amount of pressure support that is also set by the clinician. In contrast to AC/VC, where each breath is a constant volume, SIMV allows for more variation in the extra breaths above the minimum respiratory rate. For example, if SIMV is set at a rate of 8 breaths/min and a tidal volume of 500 mL with a pressure support of 5 cmH_2O, then if the patient chooses to breathe 10 times a minute over the set rate, they will breathe 18 times/min, eight of which will be guaranteed at tidal volumes of 500 mL with the remainder of varying tidal volumes on pressure support of 5 cmH_2O. "Synchronized" refers to the machine's ability to inhibit delivering a machine breath when it senses a patient-triggered breath starting, thus minimizing uncomfortable dyssynchrony.

Neonates are frequently ventilated on SIMV as a primary ventilation strategy. In pediatric and adult ventilation, both SIMV and PS are commonly used when weaning patients from the ventilator, with no data currently supporting significant differences in outcome based on ventilator mode choice between the two [20].

Adaptive Support Ventilation

Adaptive support ventilation, or ASV, is a relatively newer option designed to optimize the patient's work of breathing by combining elements of the modes discussed earlier to adjust to the patient automatically. The clinician sets four variables: FiO_2, PEEP, target minute ventilation, and high-pressure alarm. The ventilator then uses a closed-loop feedback program to adjust the respiratory rate, inspiration-expiration (I:E) ratio, and tidal volume to achieve the most efficient work of breathing. To accomplish this, ASV alternates automatically between different modes. If the patient's respiratory rate is higher than a goal, it uses PSV; if the patient is apneic, it uses AC; and if the patient's respiratory rate is lower than a goal, it uses SIMV [21].

The downsides of ASV mode include that it is only available on certain newer ventilators, it has limited data in pediatric patients, and it does not allow close control over tidal volumes.

Airway Pressure Release Ventilation

APRV is a pressure-controlled intermittent mandatory ventilation mode that can be considered an extended recruitment maneuver that encourages spontaneous respiration with brief reprieves of pressure to allow carbon dioxide exchange. It reverses the typical ratio of shorter inspiratory time and longer expiratory time, which results in the patient spending most of their time in a peak inspiration-like existence. Its terminology and concept differ considerably from the modes of ventilation discussed previously. APRV maintains a nearly constant high-pressure "open-lung" state for most of the respiratory cycle but is punctuated by brief, time-cycled releases to lower pressure. This effectively improves alveolar recruitment and oxygenation to minimize dynamic strain and with a goal of reducing ventilatory-associated lung injury (VILI). Historically, it has primarily been thought of as a rescue therapy for patients who are difficult to oxygenate, such as those with severe acute respiratory distress syndrome (ARDS) [22].

Let's walk through the nomenclature: The highest level of pressure applied, and the pressure at which most of the respiratory cycle is spent, is called P-high and is set by the clinician, typically at the desired or previous mean airway pressure. The clinician also sets the time spent at P-high, which is termed T-high, and this is typically a duration of 3–8 s, which achieves a respiratory rate of no more than 8–12 breaths/min [23]. P-low, which is typically set at 0 cm H_2O, describes the low-pressure setting to which the patient is intermittently, briefly, dropped down from P-high to allow for carbon dioxide release. The time spent at P-low is called T-low. T-low is quite brief, anywhere from 0.3 to 1.5 s. Remember, there typically is no PEEP in APRV as P-low is usually set to 0 cm H_2O—so how is it possible that the patient does not significantly derecruit when dropped from P-high? Targeting the time it takes for the patient to partly but not fully exhale helps maintain alveolar recruitment, essentially using the patient's auto-PEEP to keep alveoli open. This time to incomplete exhalation is obtained by setting T-low to the time needed for the peak expiratory flow rate (PEFR) to reach about 50% (although between 25% and 75% may be used). This essentially guarantees that airway pressures never reach zero and recruitment is maintained. During these vacillations between P-high and P-low, the patient is allowed to breathe spontaneously, which further facilitates gas exchange and alveolar recruitment [24]. Figure 6.7 shows a transport ventilator using APRV.

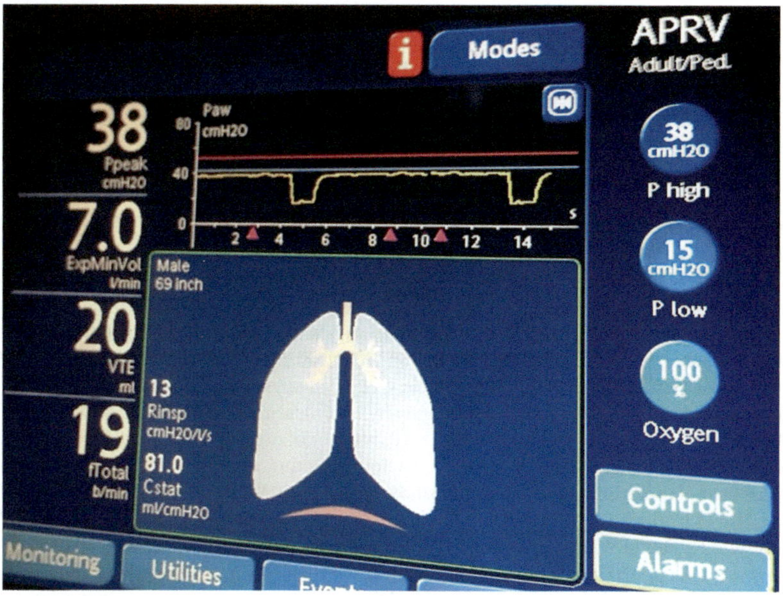

Fig. 6.7 This transport ventilator shows APRV. These settings are atypical, as the P-high is 38 cmH_2O, significantly above 30 cmH_2O. Additionally, the P-low is usually 0, but in this case, it was set at 15 cmH_2O. This photo thus represents a patient in extremis who was on very high pressures to try to maintain oxygenation

Important considerations with APRV include monitoring for significant cardiovascular implications given the increased intrathoracic pressure. The short expiratory times are not tolerated in severe bronchospasm, and the high pressures are not appropriate for those with recent pulmonary resection or those with severe restrictive lung disease. Additionally, this ventilation mode tends to lead to some degree of hypercarbia [25].

References

1. Bazuaye EA, Stone TN, Corris PA, Gibson GJ. Variability of inspired oxygen concentration with nasal cannulas. Thorax. 1992;47(8):609–11. https://doi.org/10.1136/thx.47.8.609.
2. Fuentes S, Chowdhury YS. Fraction of inspired oxygen. Treasure Island: StatPearls Publishing LLC; 2022.
3. Markovitz GH, Colthurst J, Storer TW, Cooper CB. Effective inspired oxygen concentration measured via transtracheal and oral gas analysis. Respir Care. 2010;55(4):453–9.
4. Tiep B. Portable oxygen therapy with oxygen conserving devices and methodologies. Monaldi Arch Chest Dis. 1995;50(1):51–7.
5. Milross J, Young IH, Donnelly P. The oxygen delivery characteristics of the Hudson Oxy-one face mask. Anaesth Intensive Care. 1989;17(2):180–4. https://doi.org/10.1177/0310057X8901700210.
6. Bateman NT, Leach RM. ABC of oxygen. Acute oxygen therapy. BMJ. 1998;317(7161):798–801. https://doi.org/10.1136/bmj.317.7161.798.

7. Batool S, Garg R. Appropriate use of oxygen delivery devices. Open Anesthesiol J. 2017;11(1):35–8. https://doi.org/10.2174/1874321801711010035.
8. Boumphrey SM, Morris EAJ, Kinsella SM. 100% inspired oxygen from a Hudson mask—a realistic goal? Resuscitation. 2003;57(1):69–72. https://doi.org/10.1016/S0300-9572(02)00436-7.
9. Driver BE, Prekker ME, Kornas RL, Cales EK, Reardon RF. Flush rate oxygen for emergency airway preoxygenation. Ann Emerg Med. 2017;69(1):1–6. https://doi.org/10.1016/j.annemergmed.2016.06.018.
10. Hayes-Bradley C, Lewis A, Burns B, Miller M. Efficacy of nasal cannula oxygen as a preoxygenation adjunct in emergency airway management. Ann Emerg Med. 2016;68(2):174–80. https://doi.org/10.1016/j.annemergmed.2015.11.012.
11. Drake MG. High-flow nasal cannula oxygen in adults: an evidence-based assessment. Ann Am Thorac Soc. 2018;15(2):145–55. https://doi.org/10.1513/AnnalsATS.201707-548FR.
12. Parke R, McGuinness S, Eccleston M. Nasal high-flow therapy delivers low level positive airway pressure. Br J Anaesth. 2009;103(6):886–90. https://doi.org/10.1093/bja/aep280.
13. Ritchie JE, Williams AB, Gerard C, Hockey H. Evaluation of a humidified nasal high-flow oxygen system, using oxygraphy, capnography and measurement of upper airway pressures. Anaesth Intensive Care. 2011;39(6):1103–10. https://doi.org/10.1177/0310057X1103900620.
14. Sun Y, Dai B, Peng Y, Tan W, Zhao H. Factors affecting FiO_2 and PEEP during high-flow nasal cannula oxygen therapy: a bench study. Clin Respir J. 2019;13(12):758–64. https://doi.org/10.1111/crj.13087.
15. Acevedo R, Fascia W, Pedley J, Kaul V. The use of non-rebreather masks on top of high-flow nasal cannula at maximal settings. Respir Care. 2021;66(10):3605381.
16. Nieman GF, Satalin J, Andrews P, Aiash H, Habashi NM, Gatto LA. Personalizing mechanical ventilation according to physiologic parameters to stabilize alveoli and minimize ventilator induced lung injury (VILI). Intensive Care Med Exp. 2017;5(1):8. https://doi.org/10.1186/s40635-017-0121-x.
17. Berbenetz N, Wang Y, Brown J, et al. Non-invasive positive pressure ventilation (CPAP or bilevel NPPV) for cardiogenic pulmonary oedema. Cochrane Database Syst Rev. 2019;4(4):CD005351. https://doi.org/10.1002/14651858.CD005351.pub4.
18. Bucher JT, Vashisht R, Ladd M, et al. Bag-valve-mask ventilation. Treasure Island: StatPearls; 2023.
19. Matusov Y, Li J, Resuello D, Mathers H, Fried JC. Use of pressure-regulated volume control in the first 48 hours of hospitalization of mechanically ventilated patients with sepsis or septic shock, with or without ARDS. J Intensive Care Soc. 2020;21(4):305–11. https://doi.org/10.1177/1751143719878969.
20. Chacko B, Peter J V, Tharyan P, John G, Jeyaseelan L. Pressure-controlled versus volume-controlled ventilation for acute respiratory failure due to acute lung injury (ALI) or acute respiratory distress syndrome (ARDS). Cochrane Database Syst Rev. 2015. https://doi.org/10.1002/14651858.CD008807.pub2.
21. Titus A, Sanghavi D. Adaptive support ventilation. Treasure Island: StatPearls Publishing LLC; 2023.
22. Swindin J, Sampson C, Howatson A. Airway pressure release ventilation. BJA Educ. 2020;20(3):80–8. https://doi.org/10.1016/j.bjae.2019.12.001.
23. Daoud EG, Farag HL, Chatburn RL. Airway pressure release ventilation: what do we know? Respir Care. 2012;57(2):282–92. https://doi.org/10.4187/respcare.01238.
24. Porhomayon J, El-Solh AA, Nader ND. Applications of airway pressure release ventilation. Lung. 2010;188(2):87–96. https://doi.org/10.1007/S00408-009-9212-0.
25. Habashi NM. Other approaches to open-lung ventilation: airway pressure release ventilation. Crit Care Med. 2005;33(Supplement):S228–40. https://doi.org/10.1097/01.CCM.0000155920.11893.37.

Pressures on the Ventilator

7

Jennifer Wheeler Powers and Zack Charest

Pressures on the Ventilator

Modern mechanical ventilators deliver *positive* pressure ventilation, the opposite of normal *negative* pressure physiologic breathing. Positive pressure ventilation allows adequate oxygenation and ventilation in the absence of effective native breathing. Given the foreign nature of positive pressure ventilation in contrast to natural negative pressure, damage to the lung tissues occurs if a mechanical breath is given using excess pressure. Mechanical ventilation aims to oxygenate and ventilate adequately while minimizing the risks of lung injury from excessive positive pressure. A ventilator provides several data points regarding pressure to help accomplish this goal. The ventilator delivers a breath based on set parameters, and following a full respiratory cycle (both inhalation and exhalation), ventilators frequently may display a pressure waveform and flow waveform with their associated numeric values (see Chaps. 2, 3, and 9). Having a clear understanding of each of these values and how they relate to the patient is a cornerstone to ensuring safe positive pressure ventilation and preventing damage to the lung.

One of the most common values the ventilator provides to give information on pressure delivered is the **peak inspiratory pressure (PIP),** which represents pressures in the entire airway system and measures both resistance and compliance. The PIP is usually displayed on the ventilator screen with each breath. The measurement is derived from the apex of the pressure curve and is displayed as a value in centimeters of water pressure (cmH_2O). A normal PIP can range from 15 to 20 cmH_2O and rise with increased resistance or decreased compliance. A key factor of resistance is the turbulence or how smooth the flow of air (laminar) is through the entire system. Increased resistance against the forward flow of a ventilator breath can result from internal factors (below the tip of the ETT to the alveoli) and external

J. W. Powers (✉) · Z. Charest
Boston MedFlight, Bedford, MA, USA
e-mail: Jennifer.Powers@bostonmedflight.org; Zack.Charest@bostonmedflight.org

© The Author(s), under exclusive license to Springer Nature Switzerland AG 2024
S. R. Wilcox et al. (eds.), *Mechanical Ventilation in Critical Care Transport*,
https://doi.org/10.1007/978-3-031-66782-4_7

factors (above the ETT and back to the ventilator). Internal factors affecting resistance include decreased airway diameter from swelling, bronchoconstriction, and foreign bodies/secretions. External factors that can increase resistance include small diameter ETT, kinked tubing, or an obstruction to the system, such as secretions.

Decreased compliance to expansion of the lungs is also a product of internal and external factors. Internal factors of respiratory system compliance include surface tension (aided by surfactant) and elastic properties of the lungs. Certain disease processes that affect the elasticity of the lung parenchyma and reduce compliance include pulmonary fibrosis, pneumonia, ARDS, and atelectasis. External factors such as increased intraabdominal pressure, increased body habitus, burns, or mechanical obstructions like a pneumothorax and tight seatbelt inhibit lung expansion and may decrease compliance.

In Fig. 7.1, the diagrams show the difference between anatomical areas responsible for increased pressures in the total system. Resistance is shown as a problem in the nonconducting and conducting airways. Low resistance means less added pressure due to more laminar flow. Increased resistance results in more pressure on the system due to decreased lumen size. Compliance is a function of the lung tissue and is affected by lung parenchyma elasticity and extrinsic factors outside of the pleura, placing pressure on the lungs, and hindering lung expansion. Increased compliance related to better elasticity and less added pressure. Decreased compliance relates to greater difficulty in expanding the lungs, increasing the total pressure in the system.

The **plateau pressure (*P*$_{plat}$)** is measured when airflow is absent at peak delivery of volume or pressure (depending on the ventilator mode), i.e., a breath hold. This value reflects the pressure delivered to the alveoli and the system's compliance. The

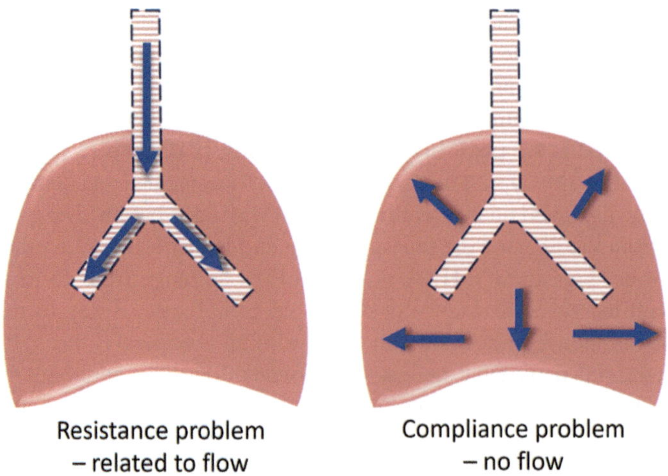

Fig. 7.1 The illustration highlights the difference between a resistance problem, related to the flow of air through the respiratory system, and a compliance problem, identified as the stiffness of the system with cessation of airflow

breath hold creates an absence of flow through the circuit and airways, which removes the resistance component of the PIP. The remaining pressure in the system describes how elastic the lungs are in proportion to the volume delivered at the inspiratory hold. The elasticity of the lungs is a result of the intrinsic and extrinsic factors discussed above, as well as the total volume delivered. To prevent alveolar injury, the P_{plat} should be maintained ≤30 cmH_2O [1]. The P_{plat} is not directly displayed on most ventilators but can be calculated by pressing the inspiratory pause button, briefly allowing all pressures to equilibrate when airflow is absent. The displayed pressure will then represent the P_{plat}.

In Fig. 7.2, we can combine all the values to examine what is happening with the patient during ventilation and retrieve data to find underlying issues. Looking at the ventilator screen, the pressure waveform is on the top, and the flow waveform is on the bottom (see Chap. 9 for further discussions on ventilator waveforms). Looking at the scale to the left of the screen, the PIP is a little over 50 cmH_2O. After pressing the inspiratory pause button, the P_{plat} is seen on the left side of the screen in the first breath on this image. The waveform is noted on the scale as 38 cmH_2O, and the calculated value is noted on the upper right-hand corner of the ventilator. Given that the P_{plat} is elevated during a breath hold, which removed the *resistance* component of PIP, this indicates that there is a *compliance* problem. The difference between the PIP and P_{plat} is greater than 5 cmH_2O, which indicates that there is *also a resistance problem*. This tracing was taken from the ventilator of a patient with end-stage COPD who developed pneumonia. These disease processes cause an increase in resistance from the decreased airway diameters resulting from bronchoconstriction and increased secretions. Pneumonia also reduces the elasticity of the lungs, causing decreased compliance. Hence, this patient has both issues—a resistance problem and a compliance problem.

To return to our diagram of resistance and compliance in Fig. 7.1, we can imagine that the patient on the left side may have a remarkably high PIP, given the increased resistance in the system. However, the P_{plat} would be low or normal with

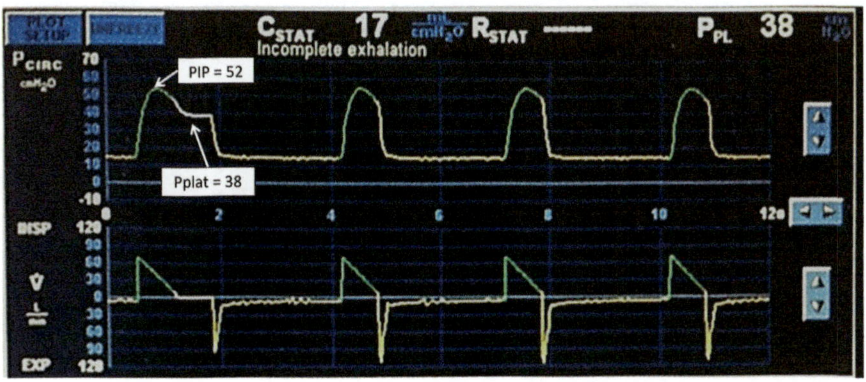

Fig. 7.2 This ventilator screen demonstrates findings in a patient with both a compliance problem (with a P_{plat} of 38 cmH_2O) and a resistance problem (with a PIP of 52, for a delta of 14 cmH_2O)

healthy lungs and normal compliance. There would likely be a large gap between the PIP and P_{plat}, confirming an issue with airway resistance. In the lungs on the right, an excess of pressure is being delivered to this system, which would increase the PIPs. In addition, the P_{plat} would also be elevated in this diagram because excess pressure is being delivered to the alveoli. To identify if resistance or compliance is the main issue, we can evaluate the difference between the elevated PIP and P_{plat} as <5 cmH_2O, indicating a compliance problem alone.

Evidence also demonstrates the importance of looking at the **driving pressure (ΔP)**. ΔP is the additive force to the alveoli, over the PEEP, delivered with each breath. The simplified calculation subtracts the PEEP from the Pplat to obtain the ΔP value [2] (Fig. 7.3). The ΔP can be described as the "hit" of the positive pressure breath on the alveolar surface. This becomes important when evaluating the safety of pressures in the system. It is generally agreed that the driving pressure should be less than 15 cmH_2O for lung protective ventilation. If the total driving pressure remains low, the alveolar "hit" is minimal, and the higher PIPs can be tolerated. The ARDS network research has gone beyond T_V and PEEP strategy as sole predictors of lung injury.

Ergotrauma is a term referring to the energy delivered to the lungs during ventilation, and it may be the most notable contributor to ventilator-acquired lung injury. Ergotrauma considers the power of the mechanical breath by evaluating the delta force (both volume and pressure) and multiplying it by each breath in a cycle. Analogous to the damage done in an aortic dissection being a factor of heart rate and blood pressure, ergotrauma demonstrates that as the frequency and force of each breath delivered to the lung increases, so does the injury to the lung tissues [3].

Another important pressure measure on the ventilator is that of the **autoPEEP** or **intrinsic PEEP (iPEEP)**. When air is trapped in the alveoli at the end of exhalation, it exerts pressure beyond the set PEEP. This pressure can be quantified on the ventilator by pressing the expiratory pause button, allowing the ventilator to equilibrate

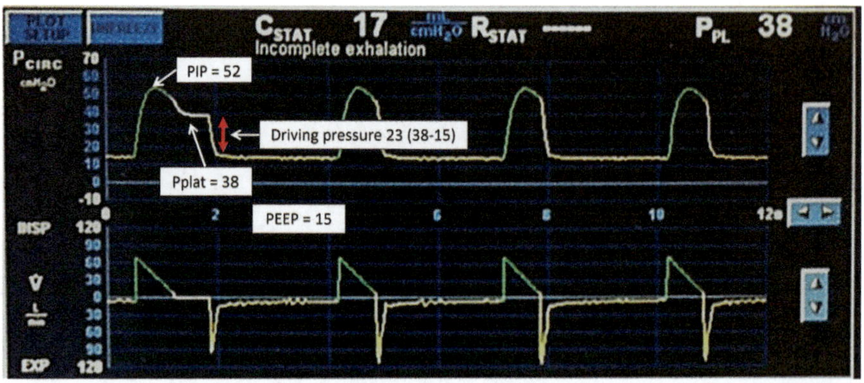

Fig. 7.3 Using the same information from Fig. 7.2, we can determine the driving pressure or the PEEP (15) subtracted from the P_{plat} (38). This driving pressure is therefore 23 cmH_2O, far greater than the goal of 15

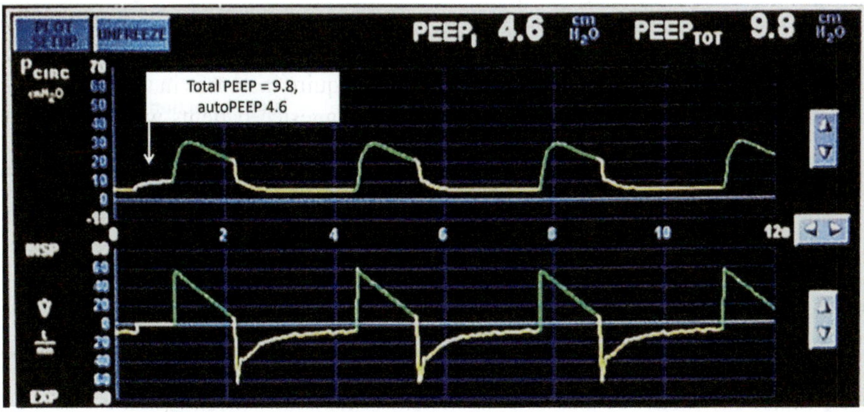

Fig. 7.4 This ventilator screen shows the total PEEP (9.8 cmH_2O) and the autoPEEP or the intrinsic PEEP (iPEEP) of 4.6 cmH_2O

the pressure at the end of expiration briefly. Like many other pressure and flow readings, many modern ventilators will show an autoPEEEP value without doing an expiratory hold.

In Fig. 7.4, the clinician has performed an expiratory hold maneuver, as noted in the first breath on this diagram. The expiratory hold calculates the total PEEP ($PEEP_{TOT}$) in the system. Assuming the clinician applied an extrinsic PEEP (ePEEP) of 5 cmH_2O, we can determine the intrinsic PEEP as follows: PEEPTOT = ePEEP + iPEEP. Therefore, iPEEP, as noted at the top of this figure, is approximately 4.6 cmH_2O. In other words, this patient is not completely exhaling at the end of each breath, leaving some additional (intrinsic) pressure in the alveoli above the set (or extrinsic) PEEP. This can also be observed in the flow tracings on the bottom of this figure, as the value at the end of each breath does not return to the baseline. This excess of pressure at the end of exhalation, as can be seen in patients with COPD, dramatically increases the work of breathing and leads to ventilator problems, such as breath stacking (see Chaps. 3, 12, and 13).

Everything discussed previously in the chapter describes measuring pressures related to ventilation and ergotrauma. The mean airway pressure (MAP), is a value that describes the average pressure in the airways over time. Higher MAP, to a point, will increase oxygenation by recruiting open alveoli and maintaining them open. MAP is a function of the pressure at inspiration and the pressure at expiration averaged based on the time at each pressure. The equation for MAP is MAP = $(PIP-PEEP) \times (T_I/T_{tot}) + PEEP$. This equation is derived for AC/PC and has some variable changes with different ventilation modes. Some modern ventilators will have this pressure already calculated.

When managing a patient with difficulty in oxygenation, ventilator changes should be aimed at increasing MAP safely. There is a point when P_{aw} becomes so high that it can overdistend the alveoli, leading to impingement of the alveolar capillary beds. This creates shunt physiology with reduced blood flow to lung areas that

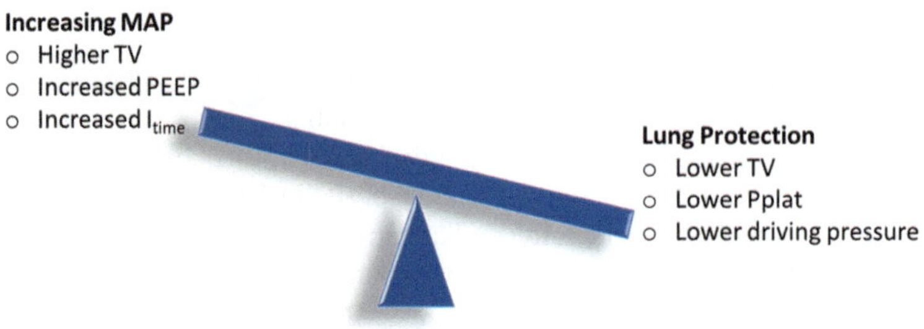

Fig. 7.5 Increasing the mean airway pressure increases oxygenation, but this benefit must be balanced against the need for lung protective ventilation

have intact gas exchange and V/Q mismatch. Calculating or recognizing where to find the value for MAP on the ventilator is also helpful when transitioning a patient between different modes of ventilation during de-escalation or escalation of care. If oxygenation is the primary concern, the MAP should be matched between ventilators to promote a safe patient transition and prevent hypoxemia and lung de-recruitment. Finding the balance between optimizing the P_{aw} to improve oxygenation while providing lung-protective ventilation is a key challenge of ventilator management (Fig. 7.5). The ventilator delivering positive pressure ventilation and the patient's airways and parenchymal tissue are independent variables that affect the pressures described on the ventilator.

The last pressure to consider is the transpulmonary pressure (P_L). The P_L parcels out the extrinsic pressures from the patient and measures the difference between the airway and pleural pressures (the pressures inside the chest but external to the lungs). This measurement requires specialized equipment to measure the intrathoracic pressure (e.g., esophageal manometry). This pressure is then subtracted from the P_{plat} or the PEEP [3]. The P_L of expiration is helpful when determining optimal PEEP strategies, and P_L of inspiration is helpful when evaluating the direct lung compliance and risk of injury. Both measurements of P_L reflect the actual pressure exerted on the alveoli during both phases of ventilation.

References

1. Malhotra A, Kacmarek R. Mechanical ventilation. In: Hagberg CA, editor. Benumof's airway management. 2nd ed. Maryland Heights: Mosby; 2007. p. 1079–122.
2. Tonetti T, Vasques F, Rapetti F, et al. Driving pressure and mechanical power: new targets for VILI prevention. Ann Transl Med. 2017;5:14. https://doi.org/10.21037/ATM.2017.07.08.
3. Grieco DL, Chen L, Brochard L. Transpulmonary pressure: importance and limits. Ann Transl Med. 2017;5(14):285. https://doi.org/10.21037/ATM.2017.07.22.

Types of Ventilators

8

Susan R. Wilcox

All mechanical ventilators have some common functions. All provide positive pressure ventilation, all provide positive end-expiratory pressure, and all provide supplemental oxygen. However, there are some differences between ICU ventilators and transport ventilators, as well as differences among types of transport ventilators. Throughout this text, we have elaborated on the mechanics of providing this ventilation, either noninvasively or inversely, highlighting various modes, or means of describing patient-ventilator interactions. Next, we will describe the ventilators themselves.

Understanding the capabilities of each type of ventilator will help clinicians know the benefits and limitations as well as help services select ventilators that are optimized for their patient populations and capabilities. A theoretical optimal device for transport would be one that is easy to use with a clear human-machine interface, lightweight, and low-cost; allows for the continuation of sophisticated ventilator modes; yet is relatively autonomous, all while offering detailed monitoring capabilities [1]. Over the last two decades, the sophistication of transport ventilators has improved dramatically, but few devices can meet all these criteria. As such, each transport organization should select the device that best suits their transport population and environment. However, the most important factor in device selection is the ability to educate and train transport clinicians on the device's capabilities and limitations. All clinicians should be facile with managing the ventilator prior to completing a transport.

At the most simplistic level, ventilation can be performed by a handbag. However, this has serious limitations, and generally, with the exception of resuscitation during cardiac arrest, manual ventilation should be avoided during transports. Mechanical ventilators offer the benefit of improved consistency in ventilation via set

S. R. Wilcox (✉)
Boston MedFlight, Bedford, MA, USA
e-mail: susan.r.wilcox@lahey.org

© The Author(s), under exclusive license to Springer Nature Switzerland AG 2024

S. R. Wilcox et al. (eds.), *Mechanical Ventilation in Critical Care Transport*,
https://doi.org/10.1007/978-3-031-66782-4_8

Table 8.1 Ventilator categories

Type of ventilator	Benefits	Challenges
Simple ventilator	• Low cost • Offers ventilator option for services that may otherwise be limited to manual ventilation	• Does not allow for titration of parameters • Not all brands offer PEEP • Few offer FiO_2 adjustments • Do not provide consistent volumes
Sophisticated ventilator	• Offers PEEP, FiO_2 titration • Waveform monitoring available	• Higher cost, may be prohibitive for some services
ICU-like ventilator	• May be used for transport for select cases, some locations (more common in Europe)	• Large • Not optimized for transport
Mass-casualty ventilator	• Sturdy, appropriate for numerous environments	• Heavy • Offer fewer ventilator settings

FiO_2 fraction of inspired oxygen, *PEEP* positive end-expiratory pressure

parameters as well as monitoring of volumes, pressures, and flow, not available with manual ventilation.

Broadly, ventilators have been divided into four categories [1, 2]. **Simple ventilators** are standard devices that deliver pressurized air but do not offer waveforms or other significant monitoring. **Sophisticated transport ventilators** offer a broader range of options for ventilation, including noninvasive ventilation and improved monitoring, usually depicting curve monitoring screens. **ICU-like ventilators** are devices that can provide all the sophisticated options available in the ICU. However, due to their size and complexity, even if they could be moved, they are not generally considered for transport on a routine basis [2]. Mass-casualty or military transport ventilators are devices dedicated for field operations. They are robust and sturdy but offer fewer monitoring capabilities [2].

The differences among the categories of ventilators are highlighted in Table 8.1. Ventilators can be divided by their means of delivering ventilation. Pneumatic ventilators use compressed oxygen for power, while turbine and compressor ventilators rely on electricity from a battery or outlet. In general, turbine and compressor ventilators are more sophisticated and offer more options than pneumatic ventilators [2].

Simple Ventilators and Mass Casualty Ventilators

Simple ventilators are quite limited in scope and capabilities. Studies have found similar characteristics between the simple and mass casualty ventilators hence they are discussed together. One study comparing transport ventilators found that fewer than half offered positive end-expiratory pressure (PEEP) valves. A majority also did not provide tidal volumes within the 10% accuracy range) even with normal respiratory mechanics [2]. The provision of a specific SpO_2 can also vary, with many using an Air-Mix blend, using the Venturi effect. The Air-Mix is a set mix of air and oxygen, distinct to each ventilator. Air-Mix varied the FiO_2 levels from 45% to 86% in a series of ventilator assessments [2]. This mechanism of blending FiO_2 can strongly impact the delivered tidal volume, with many ventilators falling far below the intended ranges [2].

Sophisticated Ventilators

For many services, sophisticated ventilators are the best option, bringing high-level ventilator settings, including noninvasive ventilation, to the transport environment. In bench testing, transport ventilators performed similarly to ICU-like ventilators with regard to tidal volume and PEEP accuracy. However, clinicians should be aware that substantial heterogeneity was found in the NIV capabilities even among sophisticated ventilators [2]. Additionally, given that sophisticated ventilators use electricity to generate pressure, the battery life is of significant importance. Figures 8.1 and 8.2 show the screens of two sophisticated ventilators with multiple capabilities and waveforms. Figure 8.3 shows another sophisticated ventilator without waveforms.

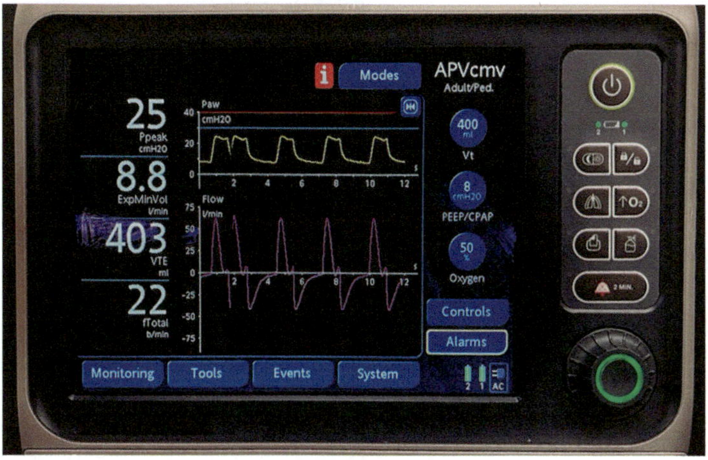

Fig. 8.1 A sophisticated ventilator demonstrating APVcmv, which is the same as assist control pressure cycled (AC/PC) in other systems. Both pressure and flow waveforms are viewed

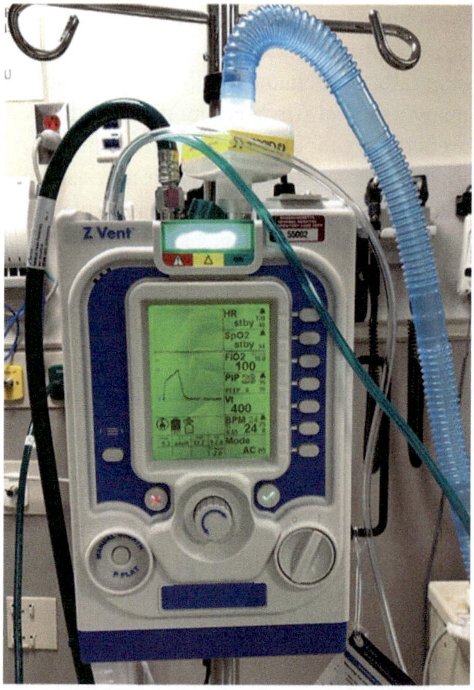

Fig. 8.2 A ventilator in AC (*v*) mode, also known as assist control, volume cycled (AC/VC), or volume control (VC) on other ventilators. The optional SpO_2 monitoring for this particular ventilator is not enabled in this photo

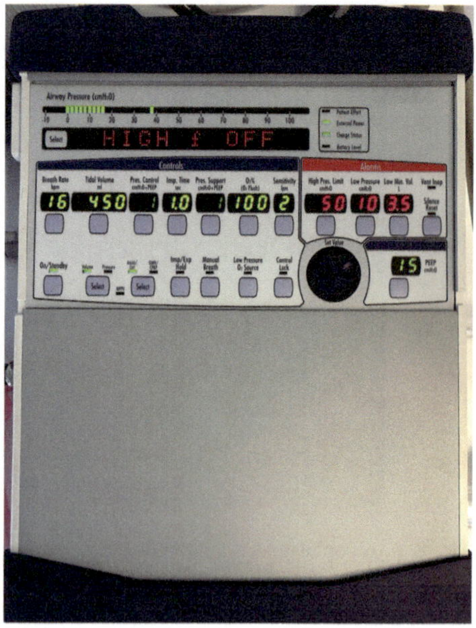

Fig. 8.3 A sophisticated ventilator that offers multiple modes of ventilation found in the ICU but does not have waveform monitoring capabilities. This ventilator is no longer in production but may still be encountered in clinical environments

ICU Ventilator Capabilities

Assessments have found major differences among the weights and volume of ventilators, impacting their ease of use in transport. Many ICU-like ventilators are not well-suited for transport and are not standard for most organizations. Some ventilators may even seem impractical for transport, given their large sizes or weights, but they are included in evaluations because they are marketed as portable [2]. As such, organizations should look closely at all specifications before deciding on a ventilator based solely on clinical capabilities. Table 8.2 demonstrates some key clinical and pragmatic differences among a selected group of ventilators. Note that no brand is endorsed, and the information available from the manufacturers varies widely.

Different Brands of Transport Ventilators

Table 8.2 highlights various brands of ventilators encountered in clinical practice.

Table 8.2 Clinical aspects of various ventilator brands

Simple and mass casualty ventilators	Technical specifications	Clinical capabilities	Notes
Oxylog 1000, Draeger (Lübeck, Germany)	Pneumatic 3.2 kg	Time-cycled, volume-controlled, and pressure-limited IPPV/CMV optional PEEP valve Fixed I:E 1:1.5 FiO2 is 100% or Air-Mix at 60%	No waveforms, compact PEEP not standard
Osiris 3, Air Liquide Medical Systems	Pneumatic 5.0 kg Battery 6–14 h	PEEP 0–15 cmH_2O FiO_2 100 or Air-Mix 70%	No waveforms
Autovent 3000, Allied Healthcare Products (Saint Louis, MO, USA)	Pneumatic 2.8 kg Operates exclusively on standard 50 psi source gas No batteries required	Allows for separate PEEP attachment	No waveforms PEEP not standard
ComPAC, Smiths Medical (Ashford, UK)	Pneumatic/compressor 11.1 kg	Driven from external gas supply or internal compressor. When driven by oxygen, FiO_2 100%, or Air-mix 45%	No PEEP 100% FiO_2, Air-mix, or air

(continued)

Table 8.2 (continued)

Simple and mass casualty ventilators	Technical specifications	Clinical capabilities	Notes
EPV200, Allied Healthcare Products (Saint Louis, MO, USA)	Pneumatic/ compressor Uses batteries to control alarms 1.4 kg Designed for mass casualty events	No PEEP Only 100% or air Allows for inspiratory time, tidal volume, and BPM controls	No waveforms Very limited in options
Sophisticated ventilators			
Elisee 350, ResMed	Turbine 4.7 kg Up to 3-h battery life	Offers pressure support as well as assist control PEEP 0–25 cmH_2O FiO_2 21–100%	Has waveforms
Monnal T60, Air Liquide Medical Systems	Turbine 3.7 kg 5-h battery life	Noninvasive and invasive ventilation PEEP 0–20 cmH_2O FiO_2 21–100%	Has waveforms
iVent 201; GE Healthcare (Cleveland, OH, USA)	Turbine 11.4 kg	Noninvasive and invasive ventilation PEEP 0–40 cmH_2O FiO_2 21–100%	Has waveforms
LTV 1200 Viasys Carefusion (San Diego, CA, USA)	Turbine 6.3 kg	Noninvasive and invasive ventilation PEEP 0–20 cmH_2O FiO_2 21–100%	No waveforms No longer in production but may remain in clinical use
T 1 Hamilton Medical (Bonaduz, Switzerland)	Turbine 6.5 kg	Noninvasive ventilation is optional, not standard Offers ASV, APRV PEEP 0–35 cmH_2O FiO_2 21–100%	Has waveforms
Oxylog 3000, Draeger (Lübeck, Germany)	Pneumatic 5.4 kg	VC-AC, VC-SIMV, Spn-CPAP and PC-BIPAP. Non-invasive ventilation with leak compensation is also provided as standard PEEP 0–20 cmH_2O FiO_2 40–100%	Has basic waveforms
Z Vent, Zoll Medical, (Chelmsford, MA, USA)	Pneumatic/ compressor 4.4 kg	AC, SIMV (optional), PS, CPAP, and Bilevel PEEP 0–30 cmH_2O FiO_2 21–100%	Has basic waveforms Allows for attachment of integrated Massimo pulse oximeter to allow SpO_2 to be displayed on the ventilator
ICU-like ventilators			
C2 Hamilton Medical (Bonaduz, Switzerland)	Turbine 9.6 kg	Noninvasive and invasive ventilation Offers ASV, APRV PEEP 0–35 cmH_2O FiO_2 21–100%	Has waveforms Has loops

(continued)

Table 8.2 (continued)

Simple and mass casualty ventilators	Technical specifications	Clinical capabilities	Notes
Servo-i Maquet Getinge (Göteborg, Sweden)	Pneumatic 20.4 kg	Noninvasive and invasive ventilation Offers NAVA, APRV FiO_2 21–100%	Has waveforms While listed as transportable, large size and weight preclude most transport
T75 Air Liquide Medical Systems (Antony, France)	Turbine 16.0 kg	Noninvasive and invasive ventilation Offers a proprietary adaptive ventilation system, APRV FiO_2 21–100%	Has waveforms
Vela Viasys Carefusion (San Diego, CA, USA)	Turbine 17.3 kg	Noninvasive and invasive ventilation PEEP 0–35 cmH_2O FiO_2 21–100%	Has waveforms

APRV airway pressure release ventilation, *ASV* adaptive support ventilation, FiO_2 fraction of inspired oxygen, *PEEP* positive end-expiratory pressure

References

1. Marjanovic N, L'Her E. A Comprehensive approach for the ergonomic evaluation of 13 emergency and transport ventilators. Respir Care. 2016;61(5):632–9. https://doi.org/10.4187/RESPCARE.04292.
2. L'Her E, Roy A, Marjanovic N. Bench-test comparison of 26 emergency and transport ventilators. Crit Care. 2014;18(5):506. https://doi.org/10.1186/s13054-014-0506-0.

Understanding the Ventilator Screen

9

Nicole King and James Boomhower

Mechanical ventilation as a treatment modality can be a complicated, often overwhelming concept. When you add in the multiple different types of ventilators on the market and the countless settings, modes, and waveforms you may encounter, understanding the mechanical ventilator screen can become even less clear (see Chap. 8 for details). However, it can be easier to interpret the different settings if you familiarize yourself with some key concepts that are universal to all ventilators (see Chaps. 2, 3, 6, and 10).

1. What are the settings?
   (a) The values set by the clinician can include the mode of ventilation (i.e., assist control vs. SIMV), the control variables (i.e., volume versus pressure), the parameters of ventilatory support (i.e., respiratory rate, inspiratory pressure, tidal volume, FiO_2, inspiratory time), and alarm/safety settings (i.e., peak inspiratory pressure (PIP), tidal volume, and/or minute ventilation limitations).
2. What is the patient's response?
   (a) For most modern ventilators, this represents values the ventilator measures regarding the patients' response to ventilation. For example, how much of the set tidal volume is being delivered to the patient? Is the patient overbreathing the set respiratory rate? Are there pressure or volume limitations being reached? If so, how do these limitations affect the patient (e.g., reaching a PIP limitation may prevent the patient from getting the full tidal volume delivered)?
3. How is this information being displayed on the ventilator screen?
   (a) Ventilators represent the patient's ventilatory status in numerical and/or graphical form. They may display information about flow, FiO_2, pressure, and volume, among other parameters.

N. King · J. Boomhower (✉)
Boston MedFlight, Bedford, MA, USA
e-mail: nicole.king@bostonmedflight.org; james.boomhower@bostonmedflight.org

© The Author(s), under exclusive license to Springer Nature Switzerland AG 2024

S. R. Wilcox et al. (eds.), *Mechanical Ventilation in Critical Care Transport*,
https://doi.org/10.1007/978-3-031-66782-4_9

(b) Some ventilators show all parameters simultaneously, but others allow the clinician to choose only one or two to display at a time.
(c) Several sophisticated ICU ventilators can represent the interaction of the patient and ventilator via waveform graphics, as described below (see Chap. 8).

Types of Waveforms

Understanding waveforms helps understand the ventilator when you have access to this information.

Scalar

Most commonly, data is viewed in the scalar format. Scalar refers to something that only has a magnitude, like volume, pressure, or flow. Scalars on the ventilator refer to the representation of the value of interest (pressure, flow, or volume) on the Y-axis graphed over time on the X-axis. These scalars provide graphical data and numerical data from the ventilator. While the numerical values and graphs can both convey similar information, such as the peak inspiratory pressure, the graphs can show consistency or variation among breaths, demonstrate synchrony (smooth, crisp waveforms, as opposed to irregular or jagged forms), and show breathing patterns. Hence, when available, clinicians should practice interpreting the numerical values and assessing the consistency of waveforms.

- *Volume-time scalar*: This represents the volume of gas delivered by the ventilator to the lungs over a period of time. This allows clinicians to see if the tidal volume is consistent and regular, as in Fig. 9.1.
- *Flow-time scalar*: This represents gas flow between the ventilator and the patient over a period of time. The scalars in Fig. 9.2 show a nice, smooth flow pattern with each breath. These waveforms can also be examined to look for ongoing

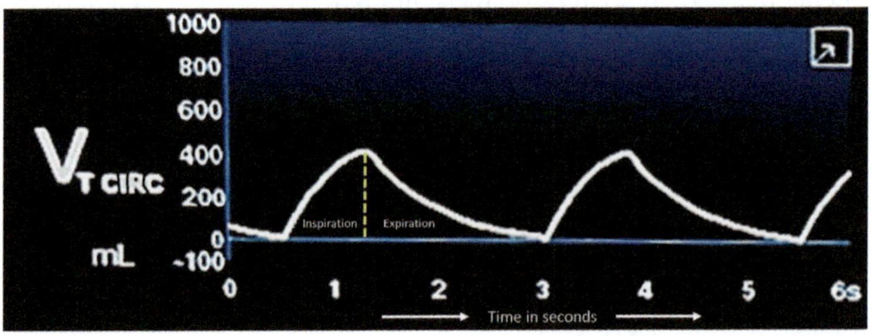

Fig. 9.1 Scalar of tidal volume over time. This represents 6 s and shows two complete cycles and one partial cycle

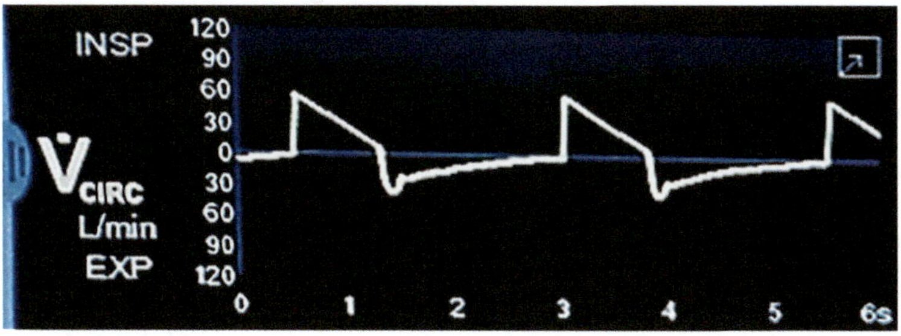

Fig. 9.2 Scalar of flow, showing 6 s. As with Fig. 9.1, it shows two complete cycles and one partial cycle. Note that the flow is smooth and regular with consistency among the waveforms

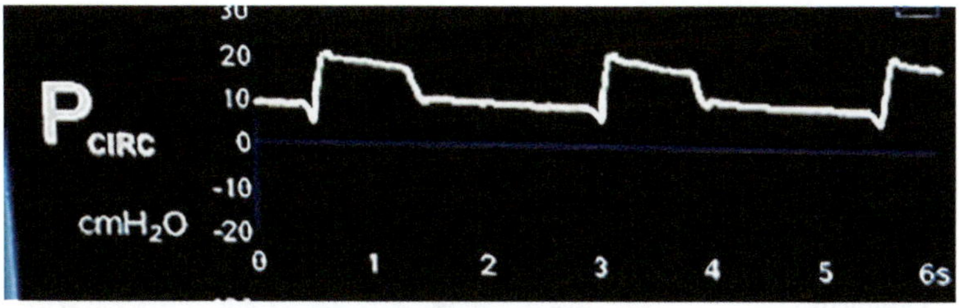

Fig. 9.3 Scalar of pressure, showing 6 s. As with Figs. 9.1 and 9.2, it shows two complete cycles and one partial cycle. There is a downward deflection with each breath, indicating a negative pressure, or an inspiratory effort from the patient

flow (the wave has not yet returned to the "0" line) when the next breath is given, indicating breath stacking.

- *Pressure-time scalar*: This represents the airway pressure over a period of time. These waveforms, as in Fig. 9.3, can show the PIP and negative deflections at the start of a breath, indicating that the patient has initiated a breath by inhaling.

Loops

Unlike scalars, loops provide the relationship between two values, usually flow and volume or pressure and volume, over time. Loops are commonly used in the ICU, and they can provide useful data. Each loop represents one breath cycle, and they repeat with each breath.

- *Flow-volume loop*: This loop represents airflow in and out of the lungs during a breathing cycle (Fig. 9.4). These loops are useful for assessing patients with flow limitations, such as obstructive disease (COPD) (Fig. 9.5), restrictive disease (pulmonary fibrosis) (Fig. 9.6), or airway obstruction.

Figure 9.7 shows an example from an actual patient's ventilator. This patient had mild COPD.

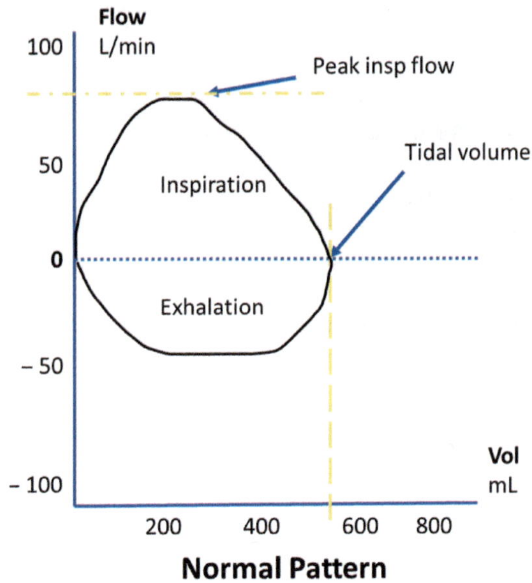

Fig. 9.4 Normal pattern for a flow-volume loop in an intubated patient. The flow and the volume are both positive in inspiration, because it is a positive-pressure ventilation. The peak inspiratory flow is about 70 L/min, and the tidal volume is about 550 mL

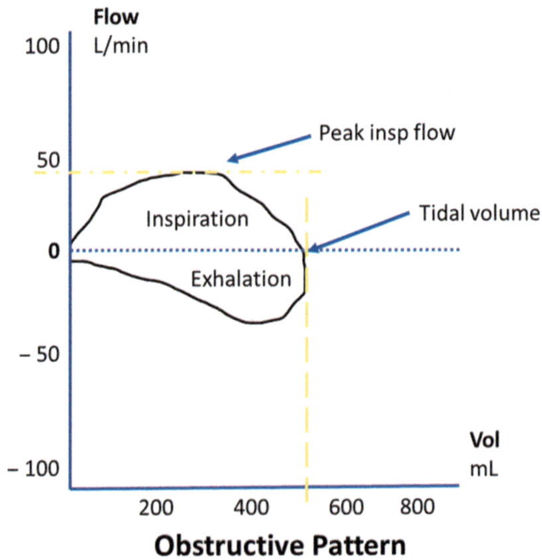

Fig. 9.5 Obstructive pattern for a flow-volume loop. The peak flow is lower, and the exhalation has a "scooped" appearance. Note that the exhalation does not come back to 0, indicating air-trapping

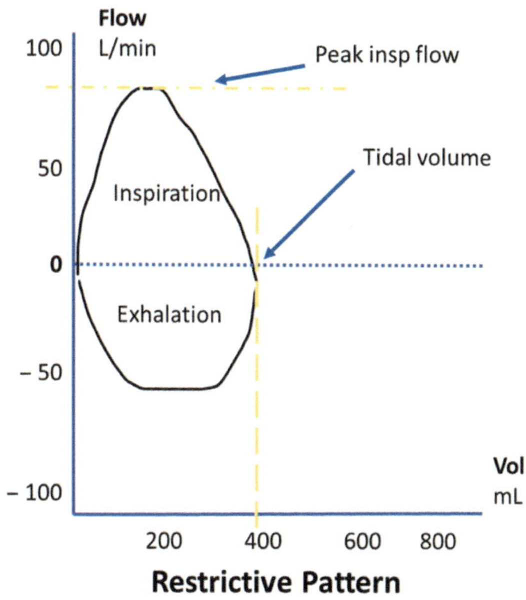

Fig. 9.6 Restrictive pattern for a flow-volume loop. The peak flow is higher, with a lower tidal volume and more forceful exhalation

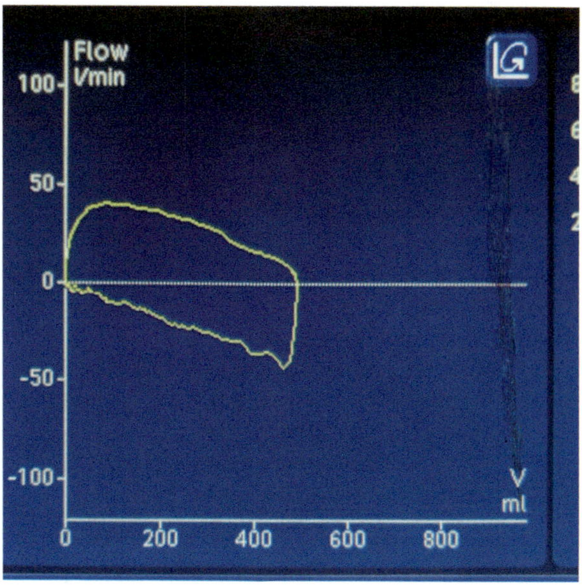

Fig. 9.7 A pattern of mild obstructive disease from a ventilator screen

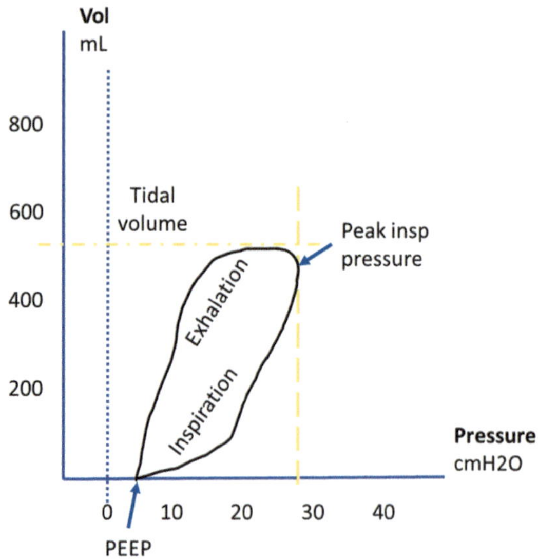

Fig. 9.8 The pressure-volume loop starts at the set PEEP (in this case, 5 cmH_2O) and the inspiratory limb increases to the peak inspiratory pressure (28 cmH_2O in this example)

- *Pressure-volume loop:* This represents the pressure in the lungs compared to the volume. These loops can be used to find inflection points under which the alveoli are collapsed, and over which, they are too distended. Figure 9.8 shows a pressure-volume loop schematic. This may help identify the level of PEEP at which the least pressure is necessary to maintain an open lung in conditions such as ARDS.

Reading Ventilator Settings

The following images show varied brands of mechanical ventilator screens with different settings and modes. While it is critical to be very familiar with the ventilator used by your organization, knowing the exact brand of the ventilator is not important to learning the key concepts of reading the ventilator screen. The more familiar a clinician is with different ventilator screens, the easier it will be to appreciate the settings and values encountered in various environments. The following photos have corresponding questions to check knowledge.

Figure 9.9 is a picture of an ICU ventilator.

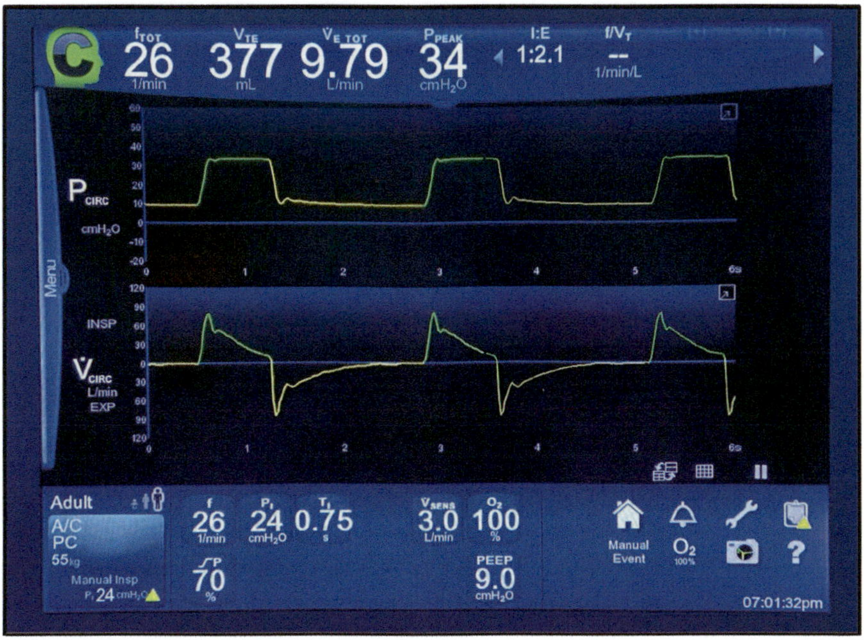

Fig. 9.9 An example of a ventilator screen in an ICU setting

1. What mode of ventilation is programmed?
2. What is the set respiratory rate? Is the patient overbreathing the ventilator?
3. What is the PEEP?
4. What is the inspiratory pressure?
5. What is the peak inspiratory pressure? How is this calculated based on the mode of ventilation?
6. What is the inspiratory time? What is the I:E ratio? How are these related?
7. What is the minute ventilation?

Answers for Fig. 9.9

1. Assist/control pressure control is denoted by the A/C PC on the screen's bottom left.
2. The RR is set at 26 b/min, seen at the bottom of the screen under the letter *f* for "frequency" of breaths. The patient is breathing 26 beats per minute in sync with the ventilator, as seen on the top left of the screen under f_{TOT}.
3. PEEP is 9 cmH_2O.
4. Inspiratory pressure, denoted by P_I on the bottom of the screen, is 24 cmH_2O.
5. The PIP/peak inspiratory pressure, denoted by P_{peak} on the top of the screen, is 34 cmH_2O. This is a combination of the PEEP and the inspiratory pressure.
6. Inspiratory time, denoted by T_I on the bottom of the screen, is 0.75 s. The I:E ratio is 1:2.1, as seen on the top of the screen. The I:E ratio is calculated as a function of the set T_I and the RR.
7. Minute ventilation, denoted by V_{eTOT} on the top of the screen, is 9.79 L/min.

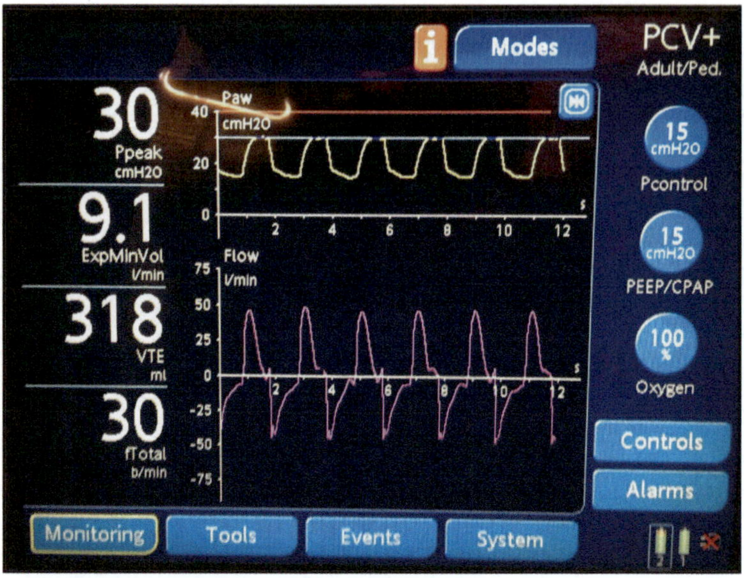

Fig. 9.10 An example of a transport ventilator screen

Figure 9.10 is a sophisticated transport ventilator.

1. What mode of ventilation is programmed?
2. What is the patient's RR?
3. What is the PEEP?
4. What is the inspiratory pressure?
5. What is the PIP?
6. What tidal volume is the patient seeing?
7. What scalars are shown on the screen?
8. Why is the pressure waveform elevated (i.e., does not touch the baseline?)

Answers for Fig. 9.10

1. Pressure control (assist control, pressure control)
2. f_{Total} is 30 breaths per minute
3. PEEP is 15 cmH_2O
4. P_{control} is 15 cmH_2O
5. P_{peak}/PIP is 30 cmH_2O
6. VTE is 318 mL
7. The top is pressure (P_{aw} = pressure airway) and the bottom is flow.
8. This is due to the high PEEP of 15. The baseline pressure is 15 cmH_2O, so the bottom of the yellow waveform starts at 15, not 0.

Figure 9.11 is another sophisticated travel ventilator.

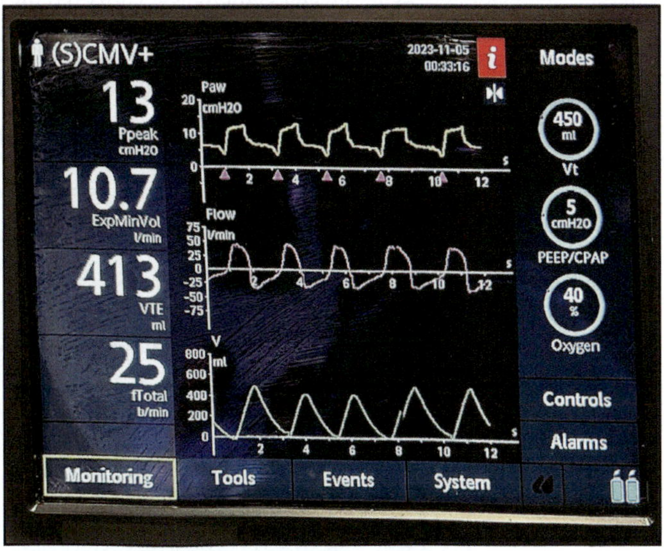

Fig. 9.11 Another example of a transport ventilator screen

1. What mode of ventilation is programmed? When is this mode typically used?
2. What are the three different waveforms on the screen?
3. What is the patient's RR? Are they overbreathing?
4. What is the PIP?
5. What is the set tidal volume? What is the patient's exhaled tidal volume?

Answers to Fig. 9.11

1. Continuous mandatory ventilation (CMV). This mode is used when the patients are deeply sedated and often paralyzed, as the ventilator provides complete control over the RR and tidal volumes delivered.
2. From top to bottom, the waveforms represent pressure, flow, and volume.
3. The patient's RR is 25 breaths per minute. Although you cannot see the set RR on this screen, you can tell that the patient is overbreathing by the small pink triangles noted underneath the waveform at the top of the screen. Each pink triangle represents a spontaneous breath.
4. The PIP/P_{peak} is 13 cmH_2O.
5. The set tidal volume (V_t) is 450 mL. The patient's exhaled tidal volume (Vte) is 413 mL. This variation in values between breaths is expected.

Figure 9.12 shows another ICU-type ventilator.

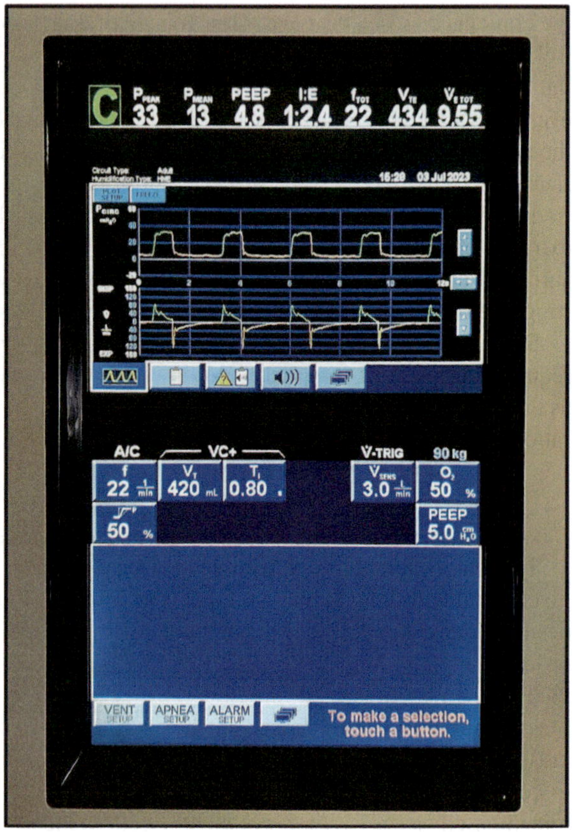

Fig. 9.12 An older ventilator screen

1. What mode of ventilation is programmed?
2. What is the tidal volume programmed versus what the patient is getting?
3. What is the trigger variable? What does this mean?

Answers to Fig. 9.12

1. Assist control volume control ventilation as denoted by A/C VC+ at the bottom left of the screen.
2. The programmed tidal volume is 420 mL, and the patient is getting 434 mL delivered. This slight variation from breath to breath is within the range of expected values.
3. The trigger variable is 3 L/min, as seen on the bottom right of the screen under VSENS. If the patient makes a spontaneous effort to breathe, the ventilator will be triggered to automatically deliver 420 mL. This is called a flow trigger. The patient can trigger the ventilator to automatically deliver a breath based on different variables such as flow and pressure. The ventilator can also be triggered to deliver a breath automatically after a certain time frame.

Figure 9.13 demonstrates another ICU ventilator.

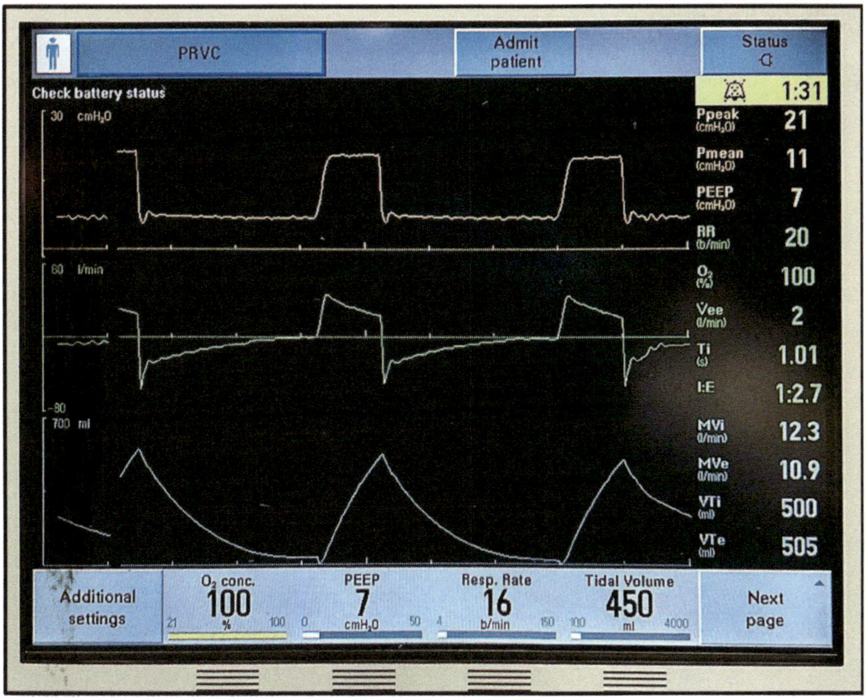

Fig. 9.13 An ICU ventilator screen

1. What mode of ventilation is programmed?
2. What is the mean airway pressure?
3. What is the set tidal volume? What is the patient's inhaled and exhaled tidal volume?
4. What is the RR? Is the patient overbreathing?

Answers to Fig. 9.13

1. PRVC: pressure-regulated volume controlled. This mode uses pressure-controlled, tidal volume-targeted breath. The ventilator delivers a breath based on multiple factors, such as lung compliance, airway resistance, and respiratory effort. Each breath is delivered with the lowest possible pressure to meet the set tidal volume.
2. The mean airway pressure (MAP), denoted as P_{mean} on the right side of the screen, is 11 cmH_2O. MAP is the average pressure applied to the airways during one ventilation cycle.
3. The set VTe is 450 mL. The patient's inhaled tidal volume (VTi) is 500 mL, and the patient's exhaled tidal volume (VTe) is 505 mL. Some variation in these values from breath to breath is normal.
4. The set RR is 16 breaths per minute, and the patient's RR is 20 breaths per minute.

Further Reading

Landry J. Ventilator waveforms and graphics made easy (overview). Respiratory therapy zone. 2023. https://www.respiratorytherapyzone.com/ventilator-waveforms/.

Landry J. Ventilator modes made easy: mechanical ventilation. Respiratory therapy zone. 2023. https://www.respiratorytherapyzone.com/ventilator-modes-practice-questions/.

Lian J, Xiong RN. Know the facts of mechanical ventilation. Nurs Crit Care. 2008;3(5):43–9. https://doi.org/10.1097/01.CCN.0000336356.61813.de.

Mechanical ventilation: pressure regulated volume control ventilation (respiratory therapy). 2023. Elsevier. https://elsevier.health/en-US/preview/mechanical-vent-pressure-regulated#ref4.

Pruitt B. Understanding ventilator basics and ventilator waveforms. Respiratory therapy. 2020. https://respiratory-therapy.com/disorders-diseases/critical-care/icu-ventilation/understanding-ventilator-basics-ventilator-waveforms/.

Wilcox SR, Aydin A, Marcolini EG. Mechanical ventilation in emergency medicine. Cham: Springer; 2022. https://doi.org/10.1007/978-3-030-87609-8.

Setting the Ventilator

10

Christine Muszalski and Kevin M. Doherty

Optimal Ventilator Settings Make the Difference

As with any medical intervention, mechanical ventilation is not without an associated risk. Choosing the appropriate ventilator settings is crucial to mitigating the damage potentially caused by mechanical ventilation in critically ill patients. Ventilator-induced lung injury occurs when the ventilator causes or aggravates a pulmonary condition and contributes to significant morbidity and mortality [1]. For example, high tidal volumes (V_t) or positive end-expiratory pressures (PEEPs) may cause high peak inspiratory pressures (PIPs), and the resultant barotrauma may promote alveolar injury and inflammation. These risks must be balanced against the necessary minimal gas exchange to support the individual patient's physiology. Conversely, low PEEPs, too, can cause excessive shearing forces on alveoli, resulting in atelectatic injury.

Suboptimal ventilator settings can adversely affect the relationships between organ systems. Standard human ventilatory physiology relies on muscle groups to expand the chest wall, which creates negative pressure to draw ambient air into the lungs via the mouth or nose. In positive pressure ventilation (PPV), the ventilator drives oxygen-enriched air into the lungs to expand the chest. During PPV, the increase in intrathoracic pressure reduces venous return from the vena cavae and may impede right ventricular function. During exhalation, the sudden decrease in intrathoracic pressure forces blood forward in circulation. This cycle of low-flow

C. Muszalski (✉) · K. M. Doherty
Boston MedFlight, Bedford, MA, USA
e-mail: christine.muszalski@bostonmedflight.org; kevin.doherty@bostonmedflight.org

© The Author(s), under exclusive license to Springer Nature Switzerland AG 2024

S. R. Wilcox et al. (eds.), *Mechanical Ventilation in Critical Care Transport*,
https://doi.org/10.1007/978-3-031-66782-4_10

and high-flow states can introduce pulmonary edema (via endothelial injury) and left ventricular dysfunction (via right ventricular dysfunction). Low minute ventilation (Ve) can exacerbate acidosis, while high Ve can result in pulmonary and cerebral vasoconstriction. It is essential that clinicians effectively resuscitate the patient, consider the physiological repercussions of PPV, and determine the optimal ventilator settings prior to initiating mechanical ventilation and adjust appropriately in response to changes in the patient.

Setting the Ventilator

Ventilator settings should be specific to the patient's underlying pathology and continuously reassessed to ensure they meet the patient's metabolic needs. Conventional teaching simplifies setting the ventilator to these modifiable parameters:

- Mode
- Tidal volume (Vt)
- Rate (*f*; frequency)
- Positive end-expiratory pressure (PEEP; EPAP in pressure-cycled modes)
- Fraction of inspired oxygen (FiO_2; expressed in %)
- Sensitivity
- Inspiratory positive airway pressure (IPAP; pressure-cycled only)
- Inspiratory time (I-time)
- Inspiratory-expiratory ratio (I:E)

Clinicians should calculate the patient's predicted body weight (PBW) to set any weight-based ventilator parameters. The size of a patient's lungs is proportional to their height, adjusted for sex, rather than body habitus or measured weight; therefore, using the patient's total body weight may cause overventilation in obese patients and underventilation in underweight patients. Clinicians previously calculated the ideal body weight (IBW) to determine weight-based parameters; however, modern respiratory studies, especially for acute respiratory distress syndrome (ARDS), champion PBW over IBW [2]. These formulae are as follows: [3]

$$\text{Males}: \text{PBW}(\text{kg}) = 50 + \left(0.91 \times \left[\text{height in cm} - 154.2\right]\right)$$

$$\text{Females}: \text{PBW}(\text{kg}) = 45.5 + \left(0.91 \times \left[\text{height in cm} - 152.4\right]\right)$$

The patient's height can also be estimated from their ulnar length, measured from the olecranon process to the olecranon process. The ulnar length is shown in a common table (Fig. 10.1):

	Ulnar Length	18.5	19.0	19.5	20.0	20.5	21.0	21.5	22.0	22.5	23.0	23.5	24.0	24.5	25.0
MALE	Height (IN)	57	58	59	59	60	61	62	62	63	64	65	65	66	67
	IBW (KG)	46	48	50	50	52	54	56	56	58	60	62	62	63	65
	Vt 5 cc/kg	232	241	251	251	260	270	279	279	289	298	308	308	317	327
	Vt 8 cc/kg	370	386	401	401	416	431	446	446	462	477	492	492	507	522
FEMALE	Height (IN)	58	58	59	59	60	60	61	61	62	63	63	64	64	65
	IBW (KG)	46	46	47	47	49	49	51	51	52	54	54	56	56	58
	Vt 5 cc/kg	228	228	237	237	245	245	254	254	262	271	271	279	279	288
	Vt 8 cc/kg	365	365	378	378	392	392	406	406	419	433	433	446	446	460
	Ulnar Length	25.5	26.0	26.5	27.0	27.5	28.0	28.5	29.0	29.5	30.0	30.5	31.0	31.5	32.0
MALE	Height (IN)	67	68	69	69	70	71	72	72	73	74	74	75	76	76
	IBW (KG)	65	67	69	69	71	73	75	75	77	79	79	81	82	82
	Vt 5 cc/kg	327	336	346	346	355	365	374	374	384	393	393	403	412	412
	Vt 8 cc/kg	522	538	553	553	568	583	598	598	614	629	629	644	659	659
FEMALE	Height (IN)	65	66	67	67	68	68	69	69	70	70	71	71	72	72
	IBW (KG)	58	59	61	61	63	63	64	64	66	66	68	68	69	69
	Vt 5 cc/kg	288	296	305	305	313	313	322	322	330	330	339	339	347	347
	Vt 8 cc/kg	460	474	487	487	501	501	514	514	528	528	542	542	555	555

Predicted Ve (normal pH): 0.1 -- 0.12 /kf IBW

Preducted Ve (Acidotic Patient): 0.15 -- 0.24 L/kg IBW

Fig. 10.1 The ulnar length, ideally measured on the left side, is a quick, noninvasive way to estimate a patient's height, thereby allowing setting the tidal volume for the predicted body weight

Mode

The first step in setting the ventilator is choosing a mode. Please see Chap. 6 for a full discussion of the modes of ventilation. As a review, mechanical ventilator modes are categorized into volume-cycled, pressure-cycled, or mixed volume-/pressure-cycled. Volume-cycled modes deliver a set tidal volume with each breath, while the pressures remain variable. Traditional volume-cycled parameters include tidal volume, respiratory rate, positive end-expiratory pressure, and the fraction of inspired oxygen (FiO_2). Conversely, a pressure-cycled mode delivers a breath to a set pressure with a variable tidal volume. Traditional pressure-cycled parameters include inspiratory positive airway pressure (IPAP), expiratory positive airway pressure (EPAP), respiratory rate (*f*), and FiO_2. The bedside clinician should determine which mode is best for the patient; however, the clinician should choose the mode with which they are most familiar, as the nuances between modes differ. There is no convincing evidence that one strategy is better than another.

Assist Control

Assist control (AC) is one of the simplest and most effective means of ventilation. It delivers a set tidal volume for every triggered breath. If the patient does not trigger the ventilator by the time another breath is indicated, per the rate set by the clinician, the ventilator will deliver a breath. AC can be set as a volume-cycled or pressure-cycled mode. In assist control, volume cycled, or commonly known as volume control (AC/VC), the patient receives a set volume with each breath. Assist control, pressure cycled, or pressure control (AC/PC) is a pressure-cycled form of A/C. Breaths are delivered to a set pressure over a set inspiratory time for each breath triggered by the patient or the ventilator.

Pressure Support

In pressure support (PS), the patient triggers every breath. The ventilator will assist the patient's respiratory effort by delivering consistent pressure (PS) while the patient inspires, and a longer inspiratory phase will result in larger tidal volumes. Additionally, the clinician sets a PEEP for this mode. This mode is commonly used to wean patients from a ventilator as they assume most of the work of breathing. As this is a spontaneous (meaning patient driven) mode of ventilation, it is often more comfortable for patients and therefore requires less sedation. However, it is an uncommon choice in the emergency setting as there is no set backup rate or tidal volume—the patient must have an intrinsic respiratory drive and cannot receive neuromuscular blocking agents.

Specialty Modes

There are a variety of specialized ventilator modes that may be beneficial for specific patient populations. Synchronous intermittent mandatory ventilation (SIMV) is similar to A/C, but the ventilator does not fully support patient-triggered breaths, rather relying on a pressure support breath (as described above). If the patient is not breathing at a predefined target rate spontaneously, the ventilator will deliver a traditional control breath as noted above. This is a common mode of mechanical ventilation for neonates to support their native respiratory rate, while minimizing sedation needs and also ensuring a minimum minute ventilation.

Pressure-regulated volume control (PRVC) combines volume- and pressure-cycle modes to deliver a set tidal volume at the lowest possible pressure calculated on a breath-to-breath basis. Volume-assured pressure support (VAPS) ventilates the patient in pressure control, but the ventilator will switch to volume control if it cannot deliver the minimum tidal volume. Airway pressure release ventilation (APRV) is a bilevel mode that ventilates via two levels of CPAP and relies on pressure changes to deliver tidal volumes [4].

Tidal Volume and Respiratory Rate

The tidal volume and respiratory rate (also referred to as frequency) should be decided in tandem because they are factors of minute ventilation as represented by the formula $Ve = Vt \times f$. The average patient's goal minute ventilation is 100 cc/kg/min PBW. Patients with significant acidosis may require increases in the target minute ventilation to 150–200 cc/kg/min PBW. It is suggested patients with significant acid-base or profound hypercarbic disturbances should be evaluated by blood gas analysis 30 minutes after significant change in ventilator settings to ensure they support the patient's physiologic needs.

Tidal volume is the air delivered into the patient's lung with each ventilation. It is a set parameter in volume-cycled modes and a variable in pressure-cycled modes (see *Inspiratory and Expiratory Positive Airway Pressures*). The goal tidal volume for the average patient is 6–8 cc/kg PBW [2]. Patients with a diagnosis of, or at risk for, acute respiratory distress syndrome (ARDS) should target tidal volumes in the 4–6 cc/kg PBW range. Larger tidal volumes of 10–12 cc/kg PBW or higher will result in elevated PIPs and may result in volutrauma.

The peak inspiratory pressure (PIP) is the highest pressure measured during the respiratory cycle and should remain <30 cmH_2O in most patients. Attempting to deliver high tidal volumes in specific pathologies (e.g., asthma, pneumonectomy) will result in critically high PIPs. Some ventilators will automatically limit tidal volumes to prevent barotrauma unless the clinician adjusts the pressure-limiting parameters. The clinician must anticipate pressure limitations when switching ventilator modes between pressure- and volume-cycled, as the ventilator may limit the delivered tidal volumes and precipitously decrease minute ventilation until the clinician can troubleshoot the issue and improve compliance/resistance.

The respiratory rate is the minimum number of breaths the ventilator provides in a minute. It is reasonable to start with a respiratory rate of 12–18 based on patient effort and then obtain a blood gas and adjust the rate and volume to achieve the minute ventilation that meets the patient's physiological needs. Modern transport ventilators have open inhalation valves, allowing the patient to breathe spontaneously over the set rate. It is generally appropriate and acceptable to tolerate this, as long as there is not associated ventilatory dyssynchrony due to breath-stacking.

For example, a clinician may elect to start a 100 kg (221 lb), 1.83 m (6 ft) patient on a tidal volume of 500 and a rate of 14:

$$Ve = Vt \times f$$

$$Ve = 500\,\text{cc} \times 14\,/\,\text{min}$$

$$Ve = 7000\,\text{cc}\,/\,\text{min}$$

This 100-kg, 1.83-m male has a predicted body weight of

$$\text{PBW}(\text{kg}) = 50 + (0.91 \times [\text{height in cm} - 154.2])$$

$$\text{PBW} = 50 + (0.91 \times [183 - 154.2])$$

$$\text{PBW} = 50 + (0.91 \times 28.8)$$

$$\text{PBW} = 50 + (26.2)$$

$$\text{PBW} = 76.2\,\text{kg}$$

This patient's goal minute ventilation is as follows:

$$Ve = 100\,\text{cc}/\text{kg}/\text{min} \times \text{PBW}$$

$$Ve = 100\,\text{cc}/\text{kg}/\text{min} \times 76.2\,\text{kg}$$

$$Ve = 7620\,\text{cc}/\text{min}$$

The patient's tidal volume is adjusted to provide 6–8 cc/kg:

$$Vt = \text{PBW} \times 6\,\text{cc}/\text{kg}$$

$$Vt = 76.2\,\text{kg} \times 6\,\text{cc}/\text{kg}$$

$$Vt = 457.2\,\text{cc}$$

$$Vt = \text{PBW} \times 8\,\text{cc}/\text{kg}$$

$$Vt = 76.2\,\text{kg} \times 8\,\text{cc}/\text{kg}$$

$$Vt = 609.6\,\text{cc}$$

Using the range of tidal volumes 460–610 cc, calculate the optimal respiratory rate:

$$Ve = Vtvf$$

$$7620\frac{\text{cc}}{\text{min}} = 550\,\text{cc} \times f$$

$$f = 13.8 =\sim 14$$

In sum, the initial ventilator settings in this 100-kg, 1.83-m patient could be set to a tidal volume of 550 cc at 14 breaths/min to achieve his goal minute ventilation of 100 cc/kg/min. If the patient's blood gas revealed an ongoing acidosis, his minute ventilation could be increased to 150–200 cc/kg/min PBW by adjusting the tidal volume (while keeping the pressures less than 30 cmH_2O) and respiratory rate as needed.

Positive End-Expiratory Pressure (PEEP)

PEEP refers to the ventilator's minimum pressure at the end of the expiratory phase. It helps maintain alveolar recruitment by keeping alveoli from collapsing and sustaining atelectatic injury. In almost every condition, it should be set to a minimum of 5 cmH_2O and slowly increased in increments of 2 cmH_2O as needed to optimize oxygenation and alveolar recruitment. Increasing the PEEP may improve their oxygen saturation and PaO_2:FiO_2 ratio if the patient has a high oxygen requirement. Patients with a body mass index >40 kg/m^2 may require additional PEEP to prevent their body habitus from derecruiting alveoli [5]. Patients with ARDS often require PEEPs >10 cmH_2O to maximize oxygenation [6]. Despite the oxygenation benefits of PEEP, the clinician should aim to keep PIPs <30 cmH_2O if possible. Increasing the PEEP may increase PIPs, especially if the patient is already overdistended. Additionally, there may come a point that further elevation in PEEP may have a negative effect on oxygenation due to this over-distension. If further increases in PEEP lead to worsening oxygenation and elevation in PIPs, it is reasonable to return the PEEP to the preceding level. Additionally, if the benefit of higher PEEP is warranted for oxygenation, the patient may require ventilation at lower tidal volumes (lower PIPs) and higher rates to avoid barotrauma.

Fraction of Inspired Oxygen (FiO_2)

FiO_2 is the percentage of oxygen delivered in each breath by the ventilator. The oxygen concentration in room air is 21%, and ventilators can provide up to 100% FiO_2 when connected to a high-flow oxygen source. Most clinicians will start at a high FiO_2 (70–100%) and titrate down to avoid unnecessary hypoxia; however, literature shows that *hyperoxia* damages the lungs and central nervous system [7]. The clinician should avoid hyperoxemia using pulse oximetry (SpO_2) to guide their initial decision-making. In the Critical Care Transport environment, a target SpO_2 of 92–94% is appropriate to titrate the FiO_2 and PEEP. Specific conditions may require different oxygenation targets, for example patients with brain injury (stroke, TBI) should avoid.

(Trigger) Sensitivity

Sensitivity adjusts the negative inspiratory flow or pressure threshold that the patient must overcome to trigger a breath. For most transport ventilators, the manufacturer applies only one type of trigger (flow or pressure). For many modern ICU ventilators, it is possible to toggle between the two types of triggers based on an individual patient's requirements, though most default to flow triggers as first line as this trigger is perceived as being more comfortable for patients. Decreasing the sensitivity of a trigger is particularly useful in transport when turbulent ground, sea, or air conditions cause the ventilator to trigger and overventilate the patient unintentionally.

For pressure triggered ventilator settings, the most common sensitivity setting is −2 cmH_2O (−0.5 to −6 cmH_2O) for trigger settings in non-neonatal ventilators The clinician can make triggering the ventilator easier for a weak patient by increasing the sensitivity to >−2 cmH_2O (i.e., less negative, closer to 0). By decreasing the sensitivity to <−2 cmH_2O (i.e., more negative, further from 0), the patient will need to expend more significant effort to trigger a breath.

Flow trigger-based mechanical ventilation detects changes in the flow rate of the continuous flow of gas through a breathing circuit (bias flow) to signal the initiation of a patient breath. This is commonly set at 1–2 l/min (0.5–20 lpm) but can be adjusted up or down based on the patient needs. Vibrations, including robust cardiac cycles, may lead to oversensing by the ventilator and deliver inappropriate breaths as the flow trigger approaches less than 1 lpm.

Inspiratory-Expiratory Ratio (I:E)

The inspiratory-expiratory ratio (I:E) is the ratio of the duration of the inspiratory and expiratory phases. Inspiration is an active process whereby the ventilator drives air into the lungs. When a cycled breath ends, the ventilator allows for passive expiration. The I:E reflects the relationship between ventilation and oxygenation, with I-time reflecting oxygenation and expiratory time (E-time) representing ventilation. Longer I-times increase mean airway pressure, which improves oxygenation. However, long I-times will always subtract from E-time, which means the patient will have less time to exhale carbon dioxide (CO_2).

This limitation can be substantial in some clinical circumstances. Suppose the patient does not fully exhale before the ventilator cycles another breath, resulting in breath stacking. In that case, pressures will build in the lungs, likely causing barotrauma, hypercarbia, and hypoxia (i.e., gas trapping, breath stacking, or Auto-PEEP). Please see Chaps. 12 and 13 for more discussion of the impacts of breath stacking.

The I:E ratio is a function of inspiratory time (I-time or flow) and respiratory rate. A homeostatic I:E is usually 1:2 to 1:5, meaning there are 2–5 s of expiration for every second of inspiration. For example, if a patient has a respiratory of 15 breaths per minute, they could have an I:E of 1:3—1 s of inspiration followed by three seconds of expiration.

Inspiratory Time (I-Time; Flow)

The I-time is how quickly the ventilator delivers its inspiratory flow or pressure. If a shorter I-time is set, the inspiratory phase will be shorter, and the I:E ratio will be longer. The ventilator will deliver the tidal volume under higher pressure in volume-cycled modes. In pressure-cycled modes, the ventilator will deliver smaller tidal volumes once it reaches the IPAP. For example, if the patient breathes 15 times/min with an I-time of 0.8 s, then the E-time will become 3.2. The I:E is 1:4.

A longer I-time will shorten the expiratory phase. If the I-time is set to 1.2 s in the same patient, their E-time will change to 2.8 s. The I:E is then 1:2.3.

Respiratory Rate and I:E

Increasing the respiratory rate increases I-time and decreases E-time. Patients who need longer expiratory phases (e.g., reactive airway disease) almost always benefit from low tidal volumes at low respiratory rates.

If the rate is set to 10 breaths/min, the patient will be ventilated once every 6 seconds. With an I-time of 1.0, the E-time would be 5.0. The I:E is 1:5.

If the rate is set to 20 breaths/min, the patient will be ventilated once every 3 s. If the I-time is set to 1.0, the E-time is 2 s. The I:E is 1:2.

Inspiratory and Expiratory Positive Airway Pressures

In pressure-cycled modes, tidal volume is a function of the inspiratory positive airway pressure (IPAP), end positive airway pressure (EPAP), inspiratory time (I-time), and the inspiratory-expiratory ratio (I:E).

IPAP and EPAP are independent variables in pressure-cycled ventilation and combine to equal the PIP (without any aggravating factors, $PIP = IPAP + EPAP$). Tidal volume is the dependent variable that changes based on the difference in pressure between IPAP and EPAP. The clinician must trend volumes and minute ventilation to ensure delivery of 6–8 cc/kg PBW and at least 100 cc/kg/min PBW, respectfully.

Setting the Ventilator: The Aftermath

In 1998, the American inventor and pitchman Ron Popeil was trying to sell rotisserie chicken ovens. He needed a catchphrase that would embody the ease and simplicity of the oven and convince consumers to purchase the niche appliance. He coined a famous phrase that survives in the American vernacular decades later: "Set it and forget it."

Clinicians cannot "set and forget" a ventilator! It is incumbent on the primary clinicians to reassess the ventilation strategy using the patient's clinical status, vital signs, lab values (primarily arterial and venous blood gases), and specialty metrics (e.g., PaO_2:FiO_2 ratio, oxygen index) to guide ventilator settings. Ventilators often require repeat adjustments to support the patient's metabolic needs as they evolve throughout their care.

References

1. Bates JHT, Smith BJ. Ventilator-induced lung injury and lung mechanics. Ann Transl Med. 2018;6(19):378–8. https://doi.org/10.21037/ATM.2018.06.29.
2. The Acute Respiratory Distress Syndrome Network. Ventilation with lower tidal volumes as compared with traditional tidal volumes for acute lung injury and the acute respiratory distress syndrome. N Engl J Med. 2000;342(18):1301–8. https://doi.org/10.1056/NEJM200005043421801.
3. Linares-Perdomo O, East TD, Brower R, Morris AH. Standardizing predicted body weight equations for mechanical ventilation tidal volume settings. Chest. 2015;148(1):73–8. https://doi.org/10.1378/CHEST.14-2843.
4. Singh PM, Borle A, Trikha A. Newer nonconventional modes of mechanical ventilation. J Emerg Trauma Shock. 2014;7(3):222–7. https://doi.org/10.4103/0974-2700.136869.

5. De Jong A, Wrigge H, Hedenstierna G, et al. How to ventilate obese patients in the ICU. Intensive Care Med. 2020;46(12):2423–35. https://doi.org/10.1007/S00134-020-06286-X.
6. Guo L, Xie J, Huang Y, et al. Higher PEEP improves outcomes in ARDS patients with clinically objective positive oxygenation response to PEEP: a systematic review and meta-analysis. BMC Anesthesiol. 2018;18(1):172. https://doi.org/10.1186/S12871-018-0631-4.
7. Mach WJ, Thimmesch AR, Pierce JT, Pierce JD. Consequences of hyperoxia and the toxicity of oxygen in the lung. Nurs Res Pract. 2011;2011:1–7. https://doi.org/10.1155/2011/260482.

Acute Respiratory Distress Syndrome (ARDS) and Hypoxemic Respiratory Failure

11

Paul S. Jansson

Definitions and Pathophysiology

Acute respiratory distress syndrome (ARDS) is an acute inflammatory lung disorder that results in diffuse alveolar damage, excessive vascular permeability, and increased lung weight that causes a loss in lung tissue available for gas exchange. ARDS may be caused by a number of different pathophysiological processes and may resemble a variety of other conditions. Classic findings for ARDS include dyspnea, hypoxemia, and alveolar infiltrates on radiographic imaging.

The diagnosis of ARDS is made by satisfying four criteria, which are referred to as the Berlin Criteria [1]. They include the following:

1. *Acute symptoms*. The onset of new or worsening symptoms must be within 1 week of a known clinical insult.
2. *Radiographic imaging*. Chest X-Ray or CT imaging must show bilateral opacities (Fig. 11.1). These opacities cannot be due to other etiologies such as atelectasis, pleural effusions, lobar collapse, or nodules.
3. *Noncardiac cause*. Because acute pulmonary edema can closely resemble ARDS, the definition of ARDS requires that the respiratory failure not be explained entirely by cardiogenic pulmonary edema or fluid overload. While pulmonary edema and ARDS can coexist, objective evaluation, such as with echocardiography, physical examination, or laboratory testing, should be used to rule out hydrostatic pulmonary edema as the primary cause of respiratory failure.

P. S. Jansson (✉)
Division of Emergency Critical Care Medicine, Department of Emergency Medicine, Brigham and Women's Hospital, Boston, MA, USA

Division of Trauma, Emergency Surgery, and Surgical Critical Care, Department of Surgery, Massachusetts General Hospital, Boston, MA, USA

Harvard Medical School, Boston, MA, USA
e-mail: pjansson@bwh.harvard.edu

© The Author(s), under exclusive license to Springer Nature Switzerland AG 2024

S. R. Wilcox et al. (eds.), *Mechanical Ventilation in Critical Care Transport*,
https://doi.org/10.1007/978-3-031-66782-4_11

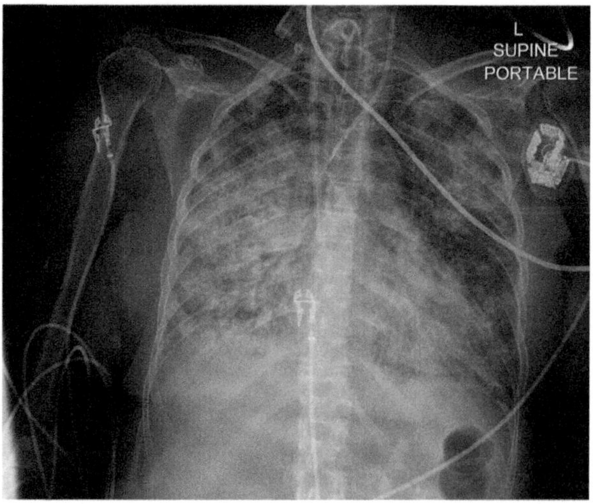

Fig. 11.1 Chest X-ray demonstrating bilateral patchy infiltrates, consistent with ARDS

4. *Hypoxemia*. The ratio between the arterial partial pressure of oxygen (P_aO_2, measured in mmHg) and the fraction of inhaled oxygen (F_iO_2, measured as a decimal; e.g., a F_iO_2 of 60% would be measured as 0.6) is used to calculate the degree of hypoxemia and must be less than 300. This measurement must be performed on at least 5 cm H_2O of positive pressure and is commonly referred to as the **P:F ratio**. The P:F ratio can be used to classify the severity of ARDS as follows:
   (a) Mild ARDS is a P:F ratio of 200–300.
   (b) Moderate ARDS is a P:F ratio of 100–199.
   (c) Severe ARDS is a P:F ratio of <100.

   A number of clinical conditions can mimic ARDS. These include pulmonary edema, bilateral pneumonia (which can also cause ARDS), inflammatory or autoimmune syndromes such as pulmonary vasculitis or acute eosinophilic pneumonia, or progressive lung diseases such as acute exacerbation of idiopathic pulmonary fibrosis or disseminated malignancy.

Pathologically, ARDS is characterized by diffuse alveolar damage to the lung tissue. Inflammation in the alveoli leads to increased capillary permeability, edema, increased extravascular lung water, and hyaline membrane formation. As the alveoli fill with fluid, they become unable to effectively participate in gas exchange, leading to shunting and, in turn, hypoxemia. After the acute phase of ARDS has passed, a fibroproliferative phase develops which may cause long-term impairment in lung functioning for some patients due to fibrosis and stiffening of the lungs [2].

Lung-Protective Ventilation

The mainstay of management in ARDS is a set of principles known as **lung-protective ventilation**, which minimizes damage to vulnerable, uninvolved portions of the lung from the ventilator. Because of their success in the management of ARDS, they have been widely adopted into the critical care setting and guide mechanical ventilation for most critically ill patients.

Low Tidal Volume Ventilation

Arguably the most important strategy in the management of patient with ARDS is the application of low tidal volume ventilation, which prevents **volutrauma**, or trauma due to high tidal volume overexpanding relatively healthy lung tissue. In a seminal trial published in *The New England Journal of Medicine*, authors from the Acute Respiratory Distress Syndrome Network (ARDSNet) compared a tidal volume of 12 mL per kilogram of predicted body weight (mL/kg PBW) to a tidal volume of 6 mL/kg PBW. The ARDSNet trial showed a decrease in mortality from 39.8% to 31.0% and an increase in ventilator-free days (12 vs. 10) in the low tidal volume group [3]. Multiple subsequent studies have verified the benefit attributable to low tidal volume ventilation [4]. This remarkable decrease in mortality led to the widespread adoption of low tidal volume ventilation to most critically ill patients at risk for ventilator-associated lung injury regardless of etiology.

The appropriate tidal volume is calculated by the patient's **predicted body weight**, not actual body weight [5]. Lung volumes vary based on patient height and sex rather than their girth. The calculation is performed as follows:

Male patients: PBW (kg) = 50 + 0.91 × (height [cm] − 152.4)

Female patients: PBW (kg) = 45.5 + 0.91 × (height [cm] − 152.4)

Note that the patient's *actual* body weight should not be used to calculate an ideal tidal volume. Once the predicted body weight is calculated, a target tidal volume of 6 mL/kg PBW is targeted, although a range of 4–8 mL/kg PBW is likely safe. Key equations are given in Table 11.1.

Figure 11.2 shows typical ventilator settings for a patient with ARDS, including low tidal volumes, higher PEEP, and an FiO_2 of 100%.

Table 11.1 Key equations

Key equations	
Predicted body weight (male) in kg	50 + 0.91 × (height [cm]−152.4)
Predicted body weight (female) in kg	45.5 + 0.91 × (height [cm]−152.4)
Minute ventilation	Respiratory rate × tidal volume
Driving pressure (no esophageal balloon)	Plateau pressure−PEEP
Driving pressure (esophageal balloon)	Plateau pressure−Esophageal pressure

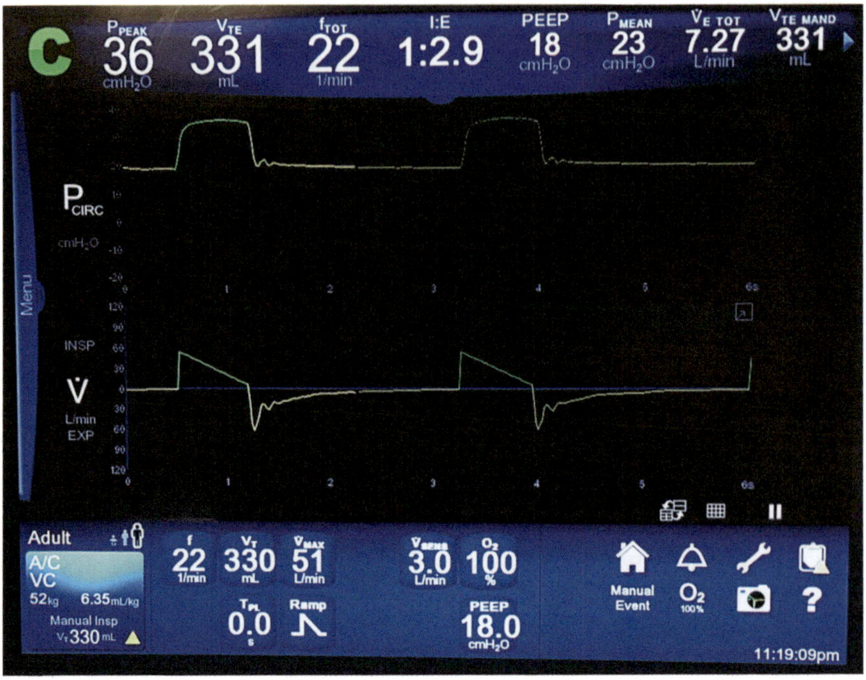

Fig. 11.2 A ventilator screen demonstrating low tidal volumes of 330 (note that the respiratory therapist entered the patient's weight, allowing the ventilator to display that this is 6.35 mg/kg of PBW.) The PEEP is 18cmH_2O and the FiO_2 is 100%, indicating that the team is having difficulty oxygenating this patient

As the patient's minute ventilation is calculated by the formula (tidal volume × respiratory rate), a decrease in the tidal volume will necessarily result in a decrease in the patient's minute ventilation unless the respiratory rate is increased. Therefore, a low tidal volume ventilation strategy will require an increase in the respiratory rate to meet the patient's requisite minute ventilation. If the respiratory rate cannot be increased enough to meet the patient's required minute ventilation, respiratory acidosis will develop. Please see Chap. 10 for a detailed discussion of the minute ventilation.

Low Plateau Pressure

After targeting a low tidal volume, the next most important concept in lung-protective ventilation is targeting a low plateau pressure (P_{plat}), which minimizes **barotrauma**, or trauma due to high pressures. A P_{plat} can be measured using the inspiratory hold feature of the ventilator, which pauses flow at the end of inspiration without allowing any expiration. The ventilator will then measure the pressure in the circuit 0.5 s after the cessation of flow, which is given as the measured P_{plat}. The P_{plat} is determined based primarily on the compliance of the lungs, which is

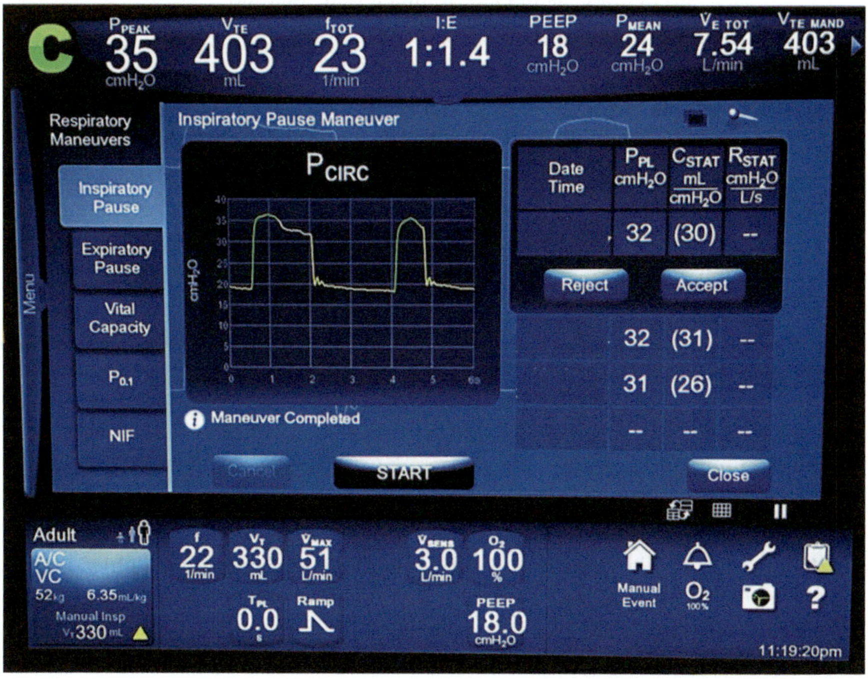

Fig. 11.3 A ventilator screen of the same patient from Fig. 11.2 demonstrating an inspiratory hold maneuver. The Pplat is 32, above the goal of 30 cmH_2O. The elevated Pplat indicates that the patient has poor compliance, a common finding in ARDS. Used with permission from Mechanical Ventilation in Emergency Medicine, second edition, 2022, Springer Nature

typically low in ARDS, and may increase, up to a point, as the positive end-expiratory pressure (PEEP) is increased.

In most situations, P_{plat} should be <30 cm H_2O to minimize barotrauma to the lungs. After setting an initial tidal volume of 6 mL/kg PBW, the P_{plat} should be checked. The settings are considered acceptable if the Pplat is <30 cm H_2O. However, if the P_{plat} is >30 cm H_2O, the tidal volume should generally be decreased, typically in 1 mL/kg increments, until the P_{plat} is <30 cm H_2O or a tidal volume of 4 mL/kg PBW is reached. It is rare for Critical Care Transport teams to be able to measure true intrapleural pressure accurately (i.e., esophageal manometry). Thus, there are some clinical situations such as super-morbid obesity, where it must be assumed that that value is elevated making the P_{plat} a less reliable surrogate marker. In these situations, it may be more acceptable (though not ideal) to have P_{plat} over 30 cm H_2O. Similar to low tidal volume ventilation, research has shown a mortality benefit from low plateau pressure ventilation [3]. Fig. 11.3 demonstrates an inspiratory hold maneuver for a patient with ARDS with an elevated Pplat.

Some patients may have severe dyssynchrony or dyspnea with low tidal volume ventilation. If increased sedation does not resolve the dyssynchrony or dyspnea, the tidal volume may increase to a tidal volume of 8 mL/kg PBW, provided that the P_{plat} remains <30 cm H_2O.

Driving Pressure

In addition to avoiding excessive tidal volumes or plateau pressures, appropriate **driving pressure**, or the difference between the plateau pressure and the level of positive end-expiratory pressure (PEEP), should be targeted. The driving pressure is another surrogate for transpulmonary pressure and reflects another marker of **barotrauma**. In general, a driving pressure of <15 cm H_2O should be targeted, although this recommendation is not supported with the same strength of evidence as that supporting a low P_{plat} [6].

Obesity and Esophageal Pressure Monitoring

In most spontaneously breathing patients, the expansion of the chest wall and elastic recoil of the lungs oppose each other to produce an intrapleural pressure, which is slightly negative at end-expiration and is increasingly negative with inspiration as the diaphragm contracts and the chest wall expands. With the shift to positive pressure ventilation, the intrapleural pressure becomes positive with the application of PEEP and increases with positive pressure inspiration. In an adult with a normal body mass index, the level of PEEP will approximate the intrapleural pressure. However, with obesity, pressure from the increased mass of the chest wall and abdominal pressure on the diaphragm will lead to increased intrapleural pressure at rest. As such, in patients with obesity, the PEEP will underestimate the intrapleural pressure. This means these patients may need higher than anticipated driving pressures and P_{plat}.

Measurement of intrapleural pressure would be invasive and is not routinely done; however, management of the esophageal pressure closely approximates the intrapleural pressure and can be used as an accurate and relatively noninvasive surrogate. Measuring an esophageal pressure with an esophageal balloon can be allowed to "adjust" for the increased intrapleural pressure when calculating the targeted P_{plat} and driving pressure [7]. When using an esophageal balloon, the targeted driving pressure is <15 cm H_2O above the esophageal pressure (rather than the PEEP) [8]. Esophageal balloons are not routinely recommended in the management of ARDS but can be utilized for patients with significant obesity for whom accurate pressures are in doubt. This procedure is inappropriate for transport but may be used at the sending or receiving hospital to optimize PEEP. Table 11.1 outlines key equations for calculating respiratory parameters.

Management of Hypoxemia

Hypoxemia is a characteristic factor of ARDS. In general, the two most effective strategies for managing hypoxemia in ARDS are adjustment of the fraction of inspired oxygen (F_iO_2) and adjustment of the positive end-expiratory pressure (PEEP).

In managing most hypoxemia, the first response is to increase the FiO_2, whether by applying supplemental oxygen or bag-valve-mask ventilation or by increasing the ventilator FiO_2. However, in ARDS, the primary mechanism of hypoxemia is from shunting of oxygen through fluid-filled and atelectatic alveoli, and therefore, increasing the F_iO_2 will typically not provide the significant increase in arterial oxygen concentration seen with other causes of hypoxemia. Therefore, while the F_iO_2 is typically set at 1.0 during the initial implementation of mechanical ventilation for ARDS, it should be lowered to target a peripheral oxygen saturation (S_pO_2) of 88–95% (P_aO_2 of 55–80 mmHg) while simultaneously adjusting PEEP to avoid oxygen toxicity.

The optimal strategy for titration of PEEP in ARDS is currently unknown. Typically, most centers use a PEEP and F_iO_2 titration strategy based on the tables used in the ARDSNet trials (Fig. 11.2). A higher-PEEP strategy may be associated with a shorter duration of mechanical ventilation [9] and is probably superior in more severe ARDS [10]. Higher levels of PEEP may recruit alveoli to participate in gas exchange, thereby decreasing shunting and improving arteriolar oxygenation. They may avoid the repetitive atelectasis-expansion-atelectasis cycle known as **atelectotrauma**. Simultaneously, higher levels of PEEP will increase intrathoracic pressure, possibly worsening hemodynamics in patients sensitive to preload reduction, and increase expiratory lung volume, placing the patient at risk of volutrauma [11]. Regardless of the titration strategy, lung-protective ventilation adherence should be paramount [12].

Decremental PEEP Titration

Many clinicians may choose to use the ARDSNet PEEP/F_iO_2 tables to dictate oxygenation strategy, but these tables do not consider individual physiology. Increasing levels of PEEP may result in the recruitment of atelectatic alveoli, therefore increasing lung compliance, but higher levels of PEEP may result in overdistension, lowering compliance and placing the patient at risk for ventilator-induced lung injury while paradoxically decreasing systemic oxygenation. A decremental PEEP titration uses the concept that oxygenation is greatest when compliance is highest and attempts to find a "best PEEP" for the patient's specific physiology.

There are several ways to determine optimal PEEP for a patient. For the Critical Care Transport team, it is important to query if "best PEEP" has been recently determined before transport and use that information to inform the PEEP titration strategy in transport. Increasing PEEP may not always be the best solution for hypoxemia in a patient with (and is set at) a "best PEEP" determined before transport. In fact, decreasing PEEP may be necessary. A slow, stepwise change in PEEP (either up or down 2 cm H_2O) no more than every 5 min allows for serial assessment of compliance and oxygenation with the change to assess for improvement (Fig. 11.4).

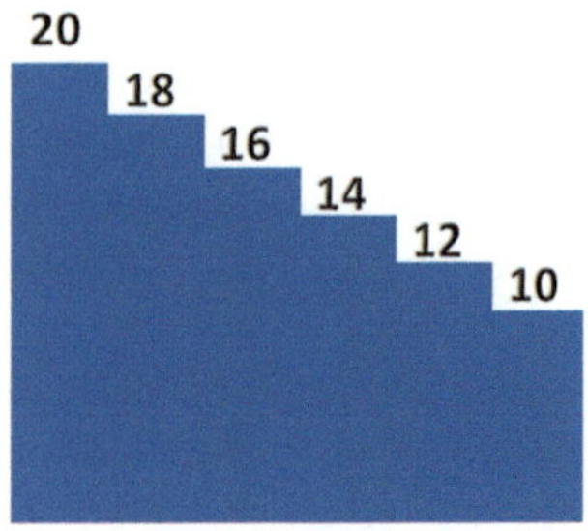

Fig. 11.4 Representation of PEEP management in a decremental PEEP trial. Used with permission from Mechanical Ventilation in Emergency Medicine, second edition, 2022, Springer Nature

Rescue Maneuvers

Some patients may have persistent hypoxemia despite appropriate titration of PEEP and F_iO_2. After ensuring that appropriate lung-protective ventilation has been achieved, the clinician has a number of strategies to "rescue" the patient from refractory hypoxemia (typically defined as a P:F of <150 mmHg).

Pharmacologic Paralysis

Neuromuscular blockade (NMB) is commonly used in severe ARDS, typically for patients with severe ventilator dyssynchrony despite adjustment of settings and optimization of sedation. NMB may decrease patient-ventilator dyssynchrony and double-triggering, including dyssynchrony not immediately apparent to the transport clinician, therefore decreasing the incidence of ventilatory-induced lung injury (Fig. 11.7). However, NMB requires higher levels of sedation. As the evidence for NMB is mixed in ICUs, it is used for selected patients in ARDS for whom the benefits are expected to outweigh the risks [13, 14]. In transport, the benefits of controlling ventilation, preventing patient movement, and thereby increasing patient safety often lead to a lower threshold for initiation of NMB and should be considered first-line "rescue" therapy for mechanically ventilated hypoxic patients in transport.

Prone Positioning

Among the most effective and evidence-based rescue maneuvers in patients with persistent hypoxemia in ARDS is the initiation of prone positioning. Figure 11.5 shows CT scan images of posterior lung derecruitment in a supine patient with ARDS. Prone positioning both improves oxygenation and decreases rates of ventilator-induced lung injury by uniform volume and lung distension [15]. Proning works through several mechanisms. First, the posterior portion of the lungs holds a large surface area. Moving the derecruited area off the posterior lungs can help recruit (Fig. 11.6). Similarly, moving the heart off the lungs helps recruit any alveoli compressed by its weight/volume. Prone positioning also relieves the abdominal pressure on the lungs. Early initiation of prone ventilation in severe ARDS decreases

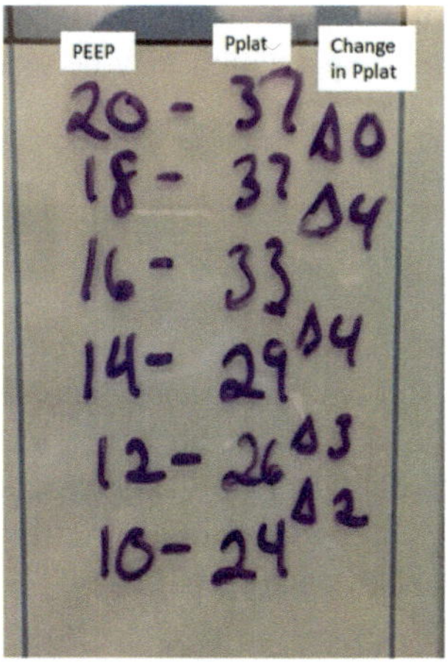

PEEP	Pplat	Driving Pressure	Compliance (TV 400mL)
20	37	17	23.5
18	37	19	21.1
16	33	17	23.5
14	29	15	26.7
12	26	14	28.6
10	24	14	28.6

Fig. 11.5 The values were taken from a BestPEEP trial. The tidal volume was steady in this trial at 400mLs, while the PEEP was adjusted. For each PEEP, the Pplat was assessed. The Pplat-PEEP then gives the driving pressure. The resultant compliance is calculated by dividing the tidal volume (400mLs) by the driving pressure. In this example, the PEEP was set 12cmH_2O. Note that at 12 of PEEP, the driving pressure is 14 and the compliance is highest, at 28.6 (same as 10cmH_2O). At 14cmH_2O, the compliance starts to decrease, indicating that the lungs may be overdistended. Used with permission from Mechanical Ventilation in Emergency Medicine, second edition, 2022, Springer Nature

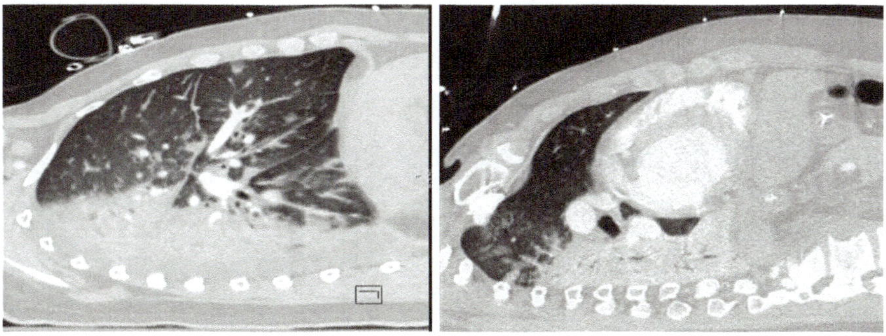

Fig. 11.6 These are two slices of a CT scan from a patient with ARDS. These images show the derecruitment that can occur along the large surface of the posterior lung, especially behind the heart. In proning the patient, this derecruitment is ameliorated and lung expansion is more uniform

mortality [16]. Patients with a P:F of <150 mmHg should undergo daily proning sessions of at least 16 h per day, absent any contraindications until oxygenation improves.

Historically, transporting patients in the prone position was uncommon, given the risks of extubation or line dislodgements. More recently, especially with the COVID epidemic, transport organizations have gained experience in transporting patients prone. This should not be undertaken lightly, as the risks are substantial.

However, the potential benefits of transporting prone, particularly when done in a planned/well-rehearsed fashion, while maintaining oxygenation may be worth the risk in select cases with significant oversight [17, 18].

Pulmonary Artery Vasodilators

Inhaled pulmonary artery vasodilators may improve oxygenation in severe ARDS by selectively dilating pulmonary vessels perfusing well-ventilated lung, thereby optimizing ventilation/perfusion matching (Fig. 11.7). Pulmonary artery vasodilators may be particularly useful in patients with preexisting pulmonary hypertension or right ventricular failure. Either nitric oxide or a prostacyclin analog (typically epoprostenol) is chosen based on institutional standard, and there is no evidence to

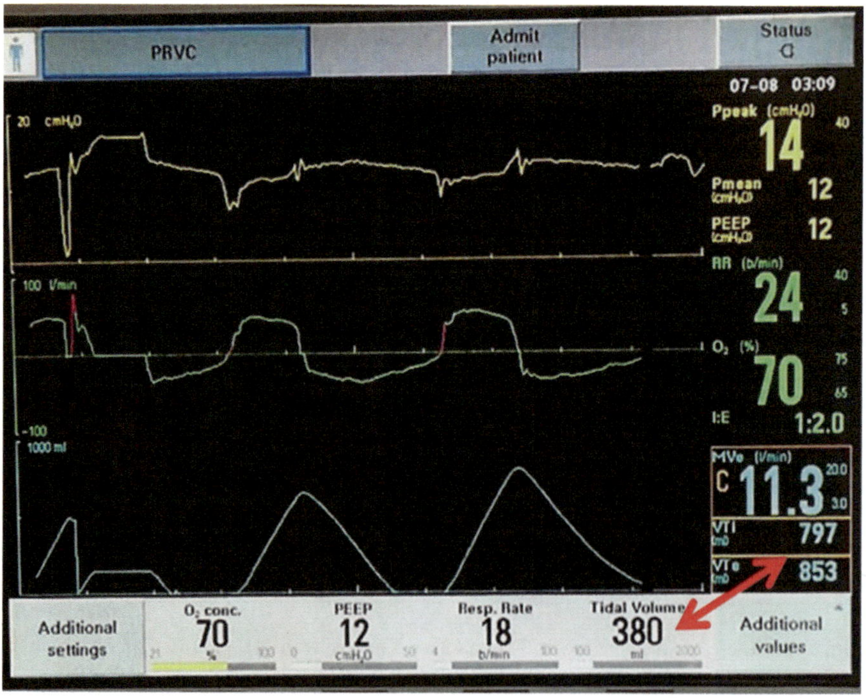

Fig. 11.7 The ventilator screen demonstrates a patient set to PRVC who has a very high respiratory drive despite sedation. Although set to low tidal volumes, the patient is taking in large volumes of ~800mLs. In this circumstance, NMB would be appropriate. Used with permission from Mechanical Ventilation in Emergency Medicine, second edition, 2022, Springer Nature

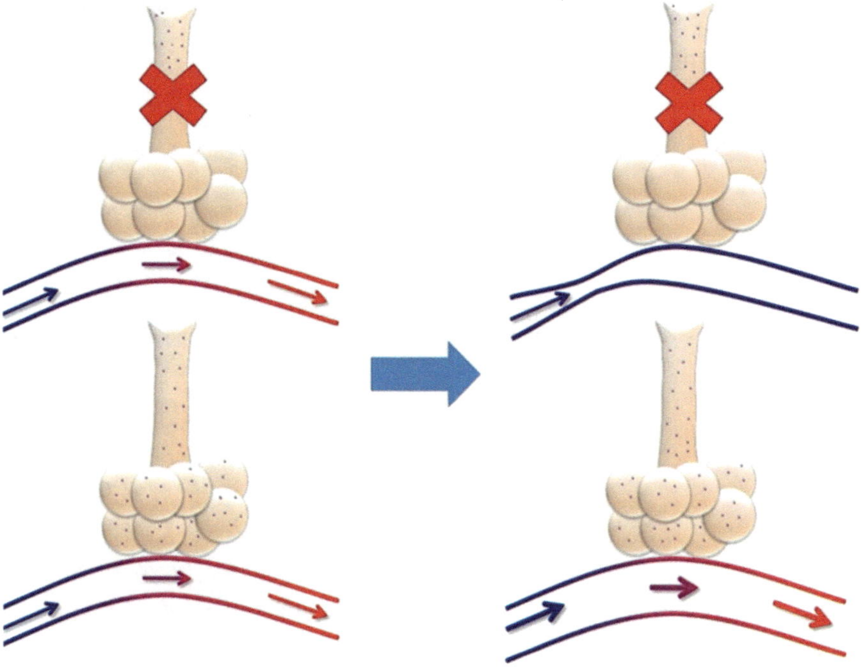

Fig. 11.8 This illustrates the concept of improved V/Q matching with inhaled pulmonary vasodilators. The vasodilator will be preferentially taken up in the preserved lung units, with resultant vasodilation, allowing more blood to flow to these areas. The portions of the lung with the most pathology (represented by the red X) will have less uptake, subsequently with less blood flow and hypoxemic vasoconstriction. Used with permission from Mechanical Ventilation in Emergency Medicine, second edition, 2022, Springer Nature

support either agent over the other. Transport with inhaled epoprostenol tends to be more pragmatic, given the compact nature and streamlined nebulization via micrometer delivery devices (Fig. 11.8). However, recent advances in inhaled nitric oxide delivery have greatly improved the ability to provide nitric oxide in transport. While the inhaled pulmonary artery vasodilators may produce a mild increase in oxygenation, there is no convincing evidence of effect on duration of mechanical ventilation, ICU length-of-stay, or mortality. Not all patients will show improvement in oxygenation with these agents, so patients should be monitored for efficacy. Patients can experience a rebound effect if a pulmonary vasodilator is stopped, so once initiated, pulmonary vasodilators should not be stopped unless under the supervision of a physician experienced in managing critically ill patients with pulmonary hypertension. Fig. 11.9 shows the setup for inhaled epoprostenol in an ICU.

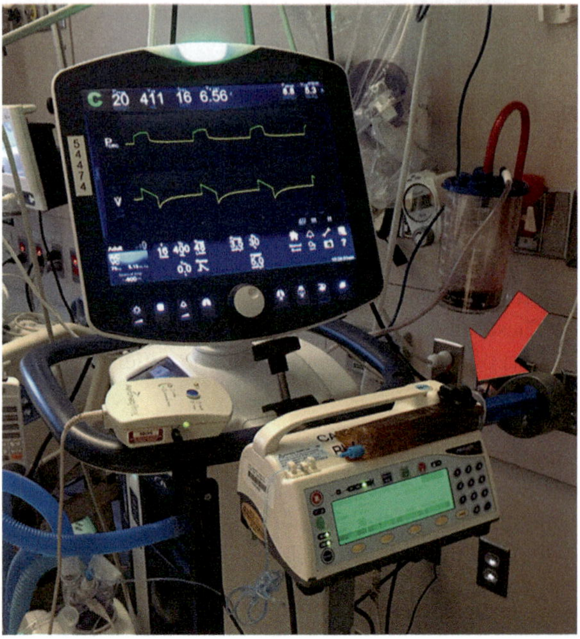

Fig. 11.9 The arrow denotes the inhaled epoprostenol, delivered to the ventilated patient by nebulization

Fluid Management

Patients with ARDS are at risk for pulmonary edema due to increased vascular permeability, even in the absence of elevated filling pressures. Targeting an even-to-negative fluid balance in patients with severe ARDS may decrease pulmonary edema and increase oxygenation. In addition to evidence showing a mortality benefit in avoiding a positive fluid balance in critically ill patients [19], a conservative fluid strategy in ARDS is associated with improved oxygenation, decreased lung injury, ventilator-free days, and ICU-free days [20]. Impact of diuresis will greatly depend on the length of transport, with minimal impact on short-duration transports (i.e., helicopter or ground) but may have a role in long-distance fixed wing missions. The decision to diurese a patient before or during transport should be made considering the patient's hemodynamics and often with medical direction. In any event, restricting fluid administration if hemodynamics allow is part of the long-term management of ARDS.

Recruitment Maneuvers

Recruitment maneuvers involve the brief application of a high level of airway pressure to expand collapsed alveoli and "recruit" them to become involved in gas exchange, thereby increasing oxygenation and compliance. However, these maneuvers increase airway pressure, risk barotrauma and pneumothorax, and increase intrathoracic pressure, reducing venous return and preload, producing hemodynamic instability. There are a number of recruitment maneuvers described in the literature and little evidence to support one over another. Common maneuvers include the brief (30–40 s) application of a high level of continuous positive pressure (30–40 cmH_2O) or stepwise increasing PEEP with a constant driving pressure or vice versa. Recruitment maneuvers are best reserved for patients with anticipated recruitable lung tissue or known derecruitment, such as in those patients who become hypoxic due to a brief disconnect from the ventilator [21].

Extracorporeal Membrane Oxygenation

Extracorporeal membrane oxygenation (ECMO) is typically the salvage therapy of last resort in severe ARDS recalcitrant to other rescue strategies. Venovenous (VV) ECMO allows oxygenation and ventilation to be maintained in the face of severe lung injury and allows for extreme lung-protective ventilator strategies to be used to minimize ventilator-induced lung injury. VV-ECMO is typically reserved for patients who are not able to oxygenate or ventilate despite optimal titration of ventilator settings (P:F < 80 mmHg), for those whom those ventilator settings are injurious and expected to produce ventilator-induced lung injury, and for those who are not a candidate for prone ventilation (Fig. 11.9). Although data on VV ECMO in severe ARDS is mixed, it is likely most beneficial when applied in experienced centers to younger patients with severe ARDS of anticipated reversible etiology with few comorbidities [22, 23] (Fig. 11.10).

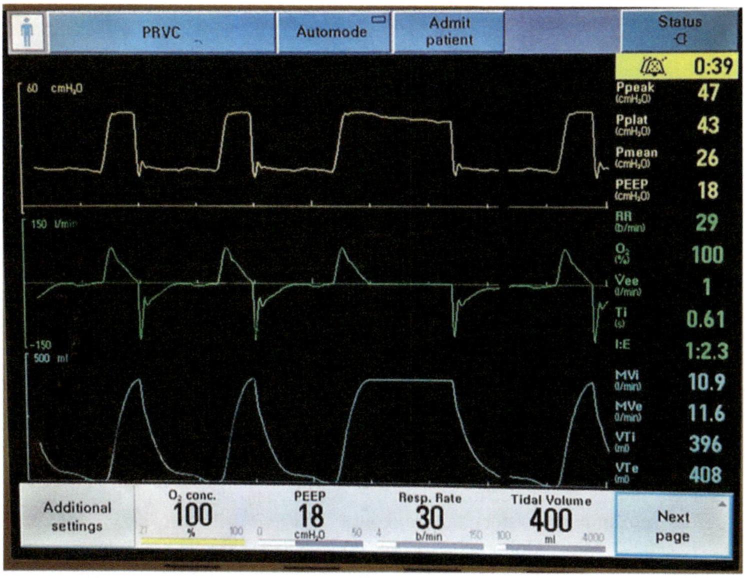

Fig. 11.10 This ventilated patient has a Pplat of 43 despite attempts at lung-protective ventilation. She was subsequently cannulated for VV-ECMO and survived. Used with permission from Mechanical Ventilation in Emergency Medicine, second edition, 2022, Springer Nature

References

1. Ranieri VM, Rubenfeld GD, Thompson BT, et al. Acute respiratory distress syndrome: the Berlin definition. JAMA. 2012;307(23):2526–33. https://doi.org/10.1001/jama.2012.5669.
2. Tomashefski JF. Pulmonary pathology of the adult respiratory distress syndrome. Clin Chest Med. 1990;11(4):593–619.
3. Acute Respiratory Distress Syndrome Network, Brower RG, Matthay MA, et al. Ventilation with lower tidal volumes as compared with traditional tidal volumes for acute lung injury and the acute respiratory distress syndrome. N Engl J Med. 2000;342(18):1301–8. https://doi.org/10.1056/NEJM200005043421801.
4. Petrucci N, De Feo C. Lung protective ventilation strategy for the acute respiratory distress syndrome. Cochrane Database Syst Rev. 2013;2013(2):CD003844. https://doi.org/10.1002/14651858.CD003844.pub4.
5. Pai MP, Paloucek FP. The origin of the "ideal" body weight equations. Ann Pharmacother. 2000;34(9):1066–9. https://doi.org/10.1345/aph.19381.
6. Amato MBP, Meade MO, Slutsky AS, et al. Driving pressure and survival in the acute respiratory distress syndrome. N Engl J Med. 2015;372(8):747–55. https://doi.org/10.1056/NEJMsa1410639.
7. Talmor D, Sarge T, Malhotra A, et al. Mechanical ventilation guided by esophageal pressure in acute lung injury. N Engl J Med. 2008;359(20):2095–104. https://doi.org/10.1056/NEJMoa0708638.
8. Baedorf Kassis E, Talmor D. Clinical application of esophageal manometry: how I do it. Crit Care. 2021;25(1):4–7. https://doi.org/10.1186/s13054-020-03453-w.
9. Mercat A, Richard JCM, Vielle B, et al. Positive end-expiratory pressure setting in adults with acute lung injury and acute respiratory distress syndrome: a randomized controlled trial. JAMA. 2008;299(6):646–55. https://doi.org/10.1001/jama.299.6.646.
10. Fan E, Del Sorbo L, Goligher EC, et al. An official American Thoracic Society/European society of intensive care medicine/society of critical care medicine clinical practice guideline: mechanical ventilation in adult patients with acute respiratory distress syndrome. Am J Respir Crit Care Med. 2017;195(9):1253–63. https://doi.org/10.1164/rccm.201703-0548ST.
11. Sahetya SK, Goligher EC, Brower RG. Setting positive end-expiratory pressure in acute respiratory distress syndrome. Am J Respir Crit Care Med. 2017;195(11):1429–38. https://doi.org/10.1164/rccm.201610-2035CI.
12. Slutsky AS, Ranieri VM. Ventilator-induced lung injury. N Engl J Med. 2013;369(22):2126–36. https://doi.org/10.1056/NEJMra1208707.
13. Papazian L, Forel JM, Gacouin A, et al. Neuromuscular blockers in early acute respiratory distress syndrome. N Engl J Med. 2010;363(12):1107–16. https://doi.org/10.1056/NEJMoa1005372.
14. National Heart, Lung and BIPCTN, Moss M, Huang DT, et al. Early neuromuscular blockade in the acute respiratory distress syndrome. N Engl J Med. 2019;380(21):1997–2008. https://doi.org/10.1056/NEJMoa1901686.
15. Menk M, Estenssoro E, Sahetya SK, et al. Current and evolving standards of care for patients with ARDS. Intensive Care Med. 2020;46(12):2157–67. https://doi.org/10.1007/s00134-020-06299-6.
16. Guérin C, Reignier J, Richard JC, et al. Prone positioning in severe acute respiratory distress syndrome. N Engl J Med. 2013;368(23):2159–68. https://doi.org/10.1056/nejmoa1214103.
17. Seethala RR, Frakes MA, Cocchi MN, et al. Feasibility and safety of prone position transport for severe hypoxemic respiratory failure due to coronavirus disease 2019. Crit Care Explor. 2020;2(12):e0293. https://doi.org/10.1097/cce.0000000000000293.
18. Boomhower J, Noland HEHE, Frakes MAMA, Seethala RRRR, Cohen JEJE, Wilcox SRSR. Transport of a nonintubated prone patient with severe hypoxemic respiratory failure due to COVID-19. Prehosp Emerg Care. 2020;25(1):55–8. https://doi.org/10.1080/10903127.2020.1819492.

19. Silversides JA, Fitzgerald E, Manickavasagam US, et al. Deresuscitation of patients with iatrogenic fluid overload is associated with reduced mortality in critical illness. Crit Care Med. 2018;46(10):1600–7. https://doi.org/10.1097/CCM.0000000000003276.
20. National Heart, Lung and BIARDS (ARDS) CTN, Wiedemann HP, Wheeler AP, et al. Comparison of two fluid-management strategies in acute lung injury. N Engl J Med. 2006;354(24):2564–75. https://doi.org/10.1056/NEJMoa062200.
21. Papazian L, Aubron C, Brochard L, et al. Formal guidelines: management of acute respiratory distress syndrome. Ann Intensive Care. 2019;9(1):69. https://doi.org/10.1186/s13613-019-0540-9.
22. Peek GJ, Mugford M, Tiruvoipati R, et al. Efficacy and economic assessment of conventional ventilatory support versus extracorporeal membrane oxygenation for severe adult respiratory failure (CESAR): a multicentre randomised controlled trial. Lancet. 2009;374(9698):1351–63. https://doi.org/10.1016/S0140-6736(09)61069-2.
23. Combes A, Hajage D, Capellier G, et al. Extracorporeal membrane oxygenation for severe acute respiratory distress syndrome. N Engl J Med. 2018;378(21):1965–75. https://doi.org/10.1056/nejmoa1800385.

Ventilator Management in Asthma

12

Elizabeth Kadow

Patients with respiratory failure from status asthmaticus who require invasive ventilatory support present a unique set of challenges when managing the ventilator. Not only do the patients tend to be quite ill when first intubated, but the management of their disease process gains complexity upon intubation, requiring careful attention to the selection and adjustment of ventilator settings.

Asthma causes reversible bronchoconstriction or narrowing of the bronchial smooth muscles (Fig. 12.1). This bronchoconstriction results in increased airway resistance particularly in the small distal airways, causing diminished airflow rates, premature closure of the airways, hyperinflation of the lungs, and decreased elasticity, resulting in air-trapping [1].

While this chapter focuses on managing the ventilator in status asthmaticus, the most important intervention in this patient population is the continual aggressive treatment of the underlying disease process. This includes the use of bronchodilators, steroids, magnesium, epinephrine, or terbutaline, as well as supportive measures such as intravenous fluids, and attention to possible precipitating causes such as pneumonia. Appropriate analgesia and sedation are also critical factors to consider. The utilization of ketamine as a sedative choice is attractive due to its inherent bronchodilatory actions via the indirect release of catecholamines from the adrenal glands. Propofol may also inhibit bronchoconstriction via smooth muscle relaxation and, thus, may also be useful.

Other pharmacologic therapy of the intubated patient with status asthmaticus may include neuromuscular blockade (paralytics) as another consideration. Neuromuscular blockade allows for control and increased predictability with ventilator management as the patient's intrinsic respiratory drive is removed from consideration. Continuous neuromuscular blockade can improve patient-ventilator

E. Kadow (✉)
Emergency Medicine, Brown University, Providence, RI, USA

Boston MedFlight, Bedford, MA, USA
e-mail: elizabeth.kadow@bostonmedflight.org

© The Author(s), under exclusive license to Springer Nature Switzerland AG 2024

S. R. Wilcox et al. (eds.), *Mechanical Ventilation in Critical Care Transport*,
https://doi.org/10.1007/978-3-031-66782-4_12

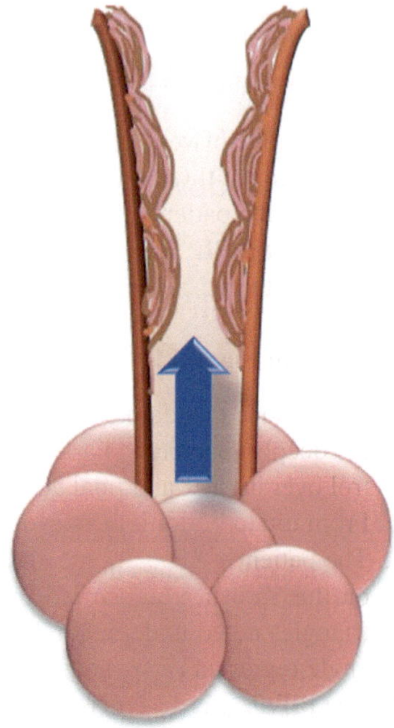

Fig. 12.1 In asthma, hyperreactivity of the smooth muscle of the bronchioles results in constriction of the airways. This results in air-trapping

synchrony, decrease breath stacking, decrease the risk of ventilator-induced lung injury, increase chest compliance, and decrease metabolic demands [2]. This is not without risks, including the risk of awareness and the need for increased sedation requirements, with possible resultant delirium [2]. It is worth noting that neuromuscular blocking agents act on the skeletal muscle, not the smooth muscle, and therefore do not actually help reverse the constriction of the smooth muscles of the bronchioles [2].

When choosing ventilator settings for patients suffering from status asthmaticus, the focus must be to allow full exhalation in order to avoid breath stacking or autoPEEP. Breath stacking occurs when some of the volume from the last breath remains because there was not enough time given for full exhalation. The persistence of exhalation is demonstrated on the ventilator by the flow waveform. In examining the flow vs. time waves, the wave showing exhalation does not return to 0 before the next breath occurs (Fig. 12.2).

Note that the magnitude of the difference from 0 does not reflect the volume or pressure of the air trapped by that breath. To quantify the pressure, the clinician performs an expiratory pause or an expiratory hold (synonyms). The expiratory pause maneuver stops all airflow at the end of exhalation, allowing pressures to equilibrate. If this pressure, the total PEEP, is above that of the set (or extrinsic) PEEP, this indicates the presence of intrinsic PEEP or autoPEEP (synonyms). This may be designated as "iPEEP" on some systems (Fig. 12.3). Breath stacking, resulting in autoPEEP, leads to lung hyperinflation, eventually causing decreased venous return and decreased cardiac output [3]. In spontaneously breathing patients, even

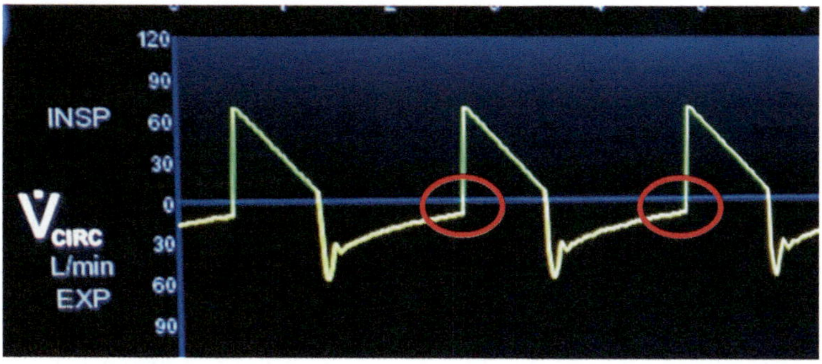

Fig. 12.2 The flow wave does not return to 0, or the baseline. This indicates that flow is still occurring when the next breath is given. Note that the delta between the line and the baseline does not quantify any values

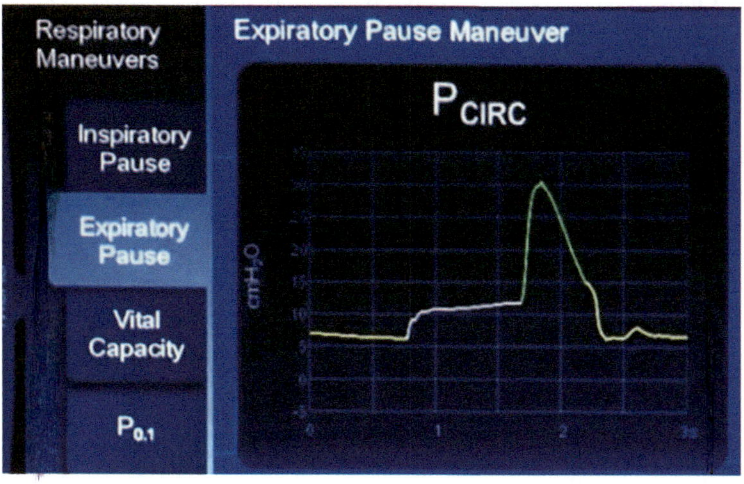

Fig. 12.3 An expiratory pause demonstrating autoPEEP or intrinsic PEEP. The total PEEP is 11cmH_2O, and the set PEEP is 5, for an autoPEEP of 6cmH_2O

those on a control mode of ventilation, the presence of autoPEEP increases the required effort for patient-initiated breaths on the ventilator, leading to dyssynchrony, distress, and increased metabolic demand. Hence, avoiding breath stacking and autoPEEP is one the most critical principles in ventilating a patient with asthma.

To allow for full exhalation, expiratory time must be maximized. For all patients, lowering the respiratory rate is the greatest way to extend expiratory time. For example, a rate of 20 breaths per minute only allows 3 seconds for a breath cycle, while a rate of 10 allows 6 s. No other intervention will be close to having such a substantial impact on the time for exhalation. Further optimizing the expiratory time will vary by the target of ventilation—either volume or pressure. For a patient in volume control, flow is the factor that is directly set. To increase the expiratory time, the clinician can increase the inspiratory flow rate, as a faster flow rate will reach the target volume sooner and allow more time in the respiratory cycle for exhalation. In pressure control, decreasing the inspiratory time or decreasing the I:E ratio will have a similar effect [3]. Ideally, patients with asthma should have a lower respiratory rate, a low I:E ratio, and a fast inspiratory flow rate leading to a shortened inspiratory time.

Minimizing the tidal volume also minimizes the time needed for exhalation, as less volume needs to be exhaled. Decreasing the respiratory rate and tidal volume reduces minute ventilation and may lead to hypercapnia and respiratory acidosis. However, permissive hypercapnia is often acceptable in this patient population to employ a lung protective ventilator strategy and avoid autoPEEP development. A pH > 7.2 is often considered acceptable, and a lower pH may be tolerated [4]. At times, well-intentioned clinicians will attempt to increase the minute ventilation to address the respiratory acidosis, but this can result in devastating increases in autoPEEP and intrathoracic pressure. Therefore, patients with respiratory acidosis from asthma should be clearly distinguished from those with metabolic acidosis requiring respiratory compensation.

When selecting initial ventilator settings in the patient with status asthmaticus, often, another parameter outside normal values will be an elevated peak inspiratory pressure (PIP). As asthma causes an increase in airway resistance, PIPs can be very elevated and at times may be even greater than 80 cmH_2O. Measurement of plateau pressure (Pplat) reflects compliance and therefore should not be elevated in most patients with asthma, unless they already have substantial air-trapping (Fig. 12.4). One can also see an elevated PIP: Pplat gradient, indicating the PIP has increased far out of proportion to the Pplat. If there is a sudden increase in Pplat, there should be concern for the development of a pneumothorax.

As the PIP may be significantly elevated, it is important to watch for several things if a patient is ventilated in a pressure control mode. The first would be

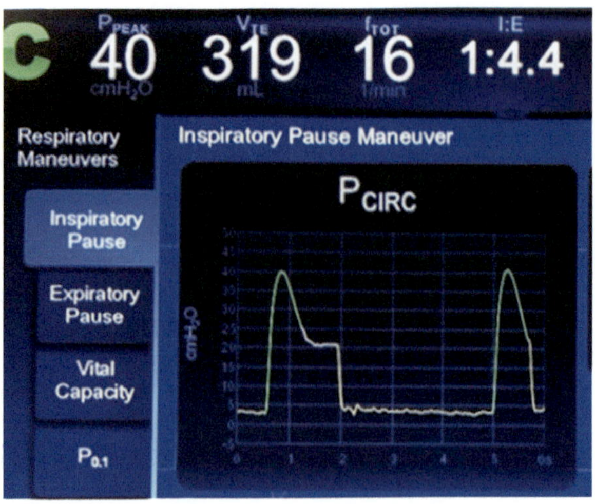

Fig. 12.4 An inspiratory pause demonstrating a PIP of 40 but a Pplat of only 20 cmH_2O

incomplete breath delivery, or insufficient tidal volume, due to a set inspiratory pressure below what is necessary for adequate ventilation. For example, if the inspiratory pressure is set for a PIP of 40 cmH_2O, but the patient requires a PIP of 60 to deliver the desired volume, there is a risk of incomplete breath delivery and hypoventilation. On the other hand, the degree of bronchospasm fluctuates with ongoing treatment of the bronchoconstriction, and the patient's PIP may also fluctuate. Setting an elevated inspiratory pressure may cause either unacceptably high tidal volumes (when the degree of bronchoconstriction is low) or low tidal volumes (when the degree of bronchoconstriction is high) [4]. Volume control ventilation offers the ability to deliver constant tidal volumes with more control over the minute ventilation compared to pressure control settings. However, as the ventilator attempts to deliver the full tidal volume, it may require pressure limits higher than other patients to do so. The pressure limits on volume control will abort a breath should it reach the pressure, regardless of the intended volume. When deciding between pressure control and volume control, it is important to understand the limitations of each setting and to frequently reassess either the volumes or pressures delivered in order to avoid barotrauma.

After selecting the initial settings, patients with asthma require close monitoring with regular blood gas monitoring to make the appropriate changes to the ventilator. Close attention should be given to ensure no autoPEEP development and the Pplat is kept <30 cmH_2O. Spontaneously breathing patients (i.e., not receiving neuromuscular blockade) who develop autoPEEP may require an *increase* in their set (extrinsic) PEEP to counteract the increased work required to initiate a breath. If it is possible to determine the level of autoPEEP, setting the extrinsic PEEP roughly at the same level should help mitigate this increased work of breathing. There is no benefit to this increase in extrinsic PEEP if the patient is receiving neuromuscular blocking agents.

With the development of autoPEEP, patients may become increasingly difficult to ventilate and develop hemodynamic instability due to decreased venous return. One difference in managing patients with asthma, as compared to most other patients, is that if the patient becomes acutely distressed, the first step is to disconnect the ventilator and assist the patient with manual exhalation by pushing gently on the chest.

In the setting of a "high pressure" alarm, if possible, one should determine if the issue is increased resistance (elevated PIP with normal Pplat) or worsening compliance (elevated Pplat). If the cause is elevated resistance, manually ventilate using a bag. If it is easy to ventilate with a bag, the issue is likely due to the ventilator or ventilator circuit itself (including obstructed filter, kinking of the circuit, etc.). If the patient is not easy to bag, the next step is to suction to remove any secretions or mucous plugs. If the patient continues to be difficult to bag, the cause is likely related to worsening bronchospasm, and efforts toward further bronchodilation should be increased [4].

If the issue is due to worsening compliance (i.e., the Pplat is elevated), the considerations should be air-trapping, pneumothorax, or developing pneumonia, ARDS, or atelectasis. The patient should then be treated for the inciting cause. In the case of air-trapping/autoPEEP, this means manual exhalation assistance by pushing on the chest after the ventilator is disconnected. The patient will then require adjustment of the ventilator settings to allow for prolonged exhalation. In the case of suspected or confirmed clinically significant pneumothorax, a needle or open thoracostomy should be performed [4].

As mentioned previously, treatments for the underlying condition should be continued during transport as it will allow for easier ventilation. Management of ventilated asthmatic patients during transport is a high-risk, complex situation that requires frequent reassessment of the patient and the ventilator.

References

1. McFadden ER. Acute severe asthma. Am J Respir Crit Care Med. 2003;168(7):740–59. https://doi.org/10.1164/RCCM.200208-902SO.
2. Mosier JM, Hypes C, Joshi R, Whitmore S, Parthasarathy S, Cairns CB. Ventilator strategies and rescue therapies for management of acute respiratory failure in the emergency department. Ann Emerg Med. 2015;66(5):529–41. https://doi.org/10.1016/J.ANNEMERGMED.2015.04.030.
3. Levy BD, Kitch B, Fanta CH. Medical and ventilatory management of status asthmaticus. Intensive Care Med. 1998;24(2):105–17. https://doi.org/10.1007/S001340050530.
4. Laher AE, Buchanan SK. Mechanically ventilating the severe asthmatic. J Intensive Care Med. 2018;33(9):491–501. https://doi.org/10.1177/0885066617740079.

COPD

13

Aaron E. Bell

Background

"Chronic obstructive pulmonary disease" (COPD) is an intentionally vague and imprecise term which is used to describe various disease processes characterized by the presence of chronic inflammation of the airways. Variants include chronic bronchitis (disease predominance in the large airways) and emphysema (disease predominance in the smaller airways and alveolar regions), either of which or in combination can lead to the development of airway obstruction. The obstruction may be partially reversible, or fixed (irreversible). Chronic bronchitis and emphysema are often regarded as independent processes, but they share common etiologic factors and are frequently encountered together in the same patient (Fig. 13.1).

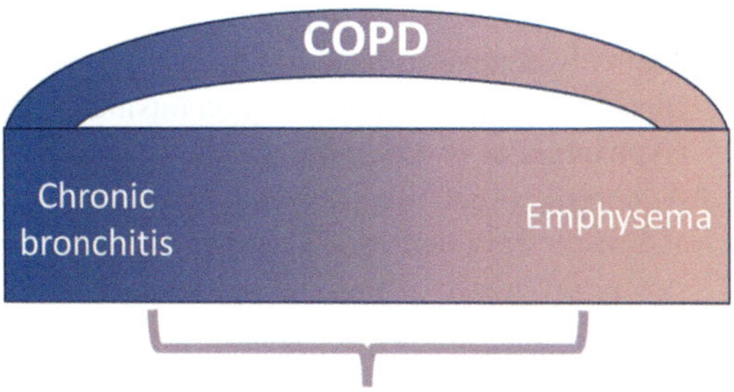

Fig. 13.1 COPD encompasses both chronic bronchitis and emphysema. Most patients with COPD have aspects of both

A. E. Bell (✉)
Boston MedFlight, Bedford, MA, USA
e-mail: aaron.bell@bostonmedflight.org

© The Author(s), under exclusive license to Springer Nature Switzerland AG 2024
S. R. Wilcox et al. (eds.), *Mechanical Ventilation in Critical Care Transport*,
https://doi.org/10.1007/978-3-031-66782-4_13

Clinical Presentation

Chronic bronchitis is defined by a clinical history of productive cough for at least 3 months out of the year for two consecutive years. Shortness of breath and airway obstruction, which can be reversible, are intermittently to continuously present. Cigarette smoking is by far the leading cause of development of the disease—as well as primary precipitant to acute exacerbations. Other inhaled irritants such as vaping, viral infections, and allergens may produce the same process. The predominant pathologic event is an inflammatory process in the airways, with mucosal thickening and hypersecretion of mucous, resulting in diffuse obstruction and heterogenous airway obstructions.

The clinical manifestations of chronic bronchitis are the results of the obstructive and inflammatory airway processes:

- Productive cough—thick, often purulent sputum due to the ongoing local inflammation and high likelihood of bacterial colonization and infection. Coughing, which is normally very effective in clearing normal airways, is much less effective due to narrower airways, as well as a greater volume and viscosity of secretions with decreased mucociliary clearance.
- Wheezing—persistent airway narrowing and mucus obstruction can produce wheezing demonstrating increased turbulence and resistance to air flowing in the distal airways, leading to noisy exhalation. This may be responsive to bronchodilators, representing a reversible component to the obstruction.
- Inspiratory and expiratory coarse crackles—due to the increased mucus production heard predominantly in larger airways during tidal breathing or with cough.
- Tachycardia—especially during exacerbations with increased work of breathing or hypoxia. If hypoxia is chronic and significant, evidence of pulmonary hypertension can result.
- Imaging—evidence of hyperinflation is typical with increased lung volumes and relatively depressed diaphragms.
- Blood gas—ventilation/perfusion mismatching is common in chronic bronchitis. Hypoxemia at rest is more profound in chronic bronchitis than in emphysema. As chronic bronchitis progresses, it is not uncommon to find an increased PCO_2 and respiratory acidosis due to decreased alveolar ventilation. If this process is slowly progressive, and kidney function is adequate, the patient may develop a compensatory metabolic alkalosis. Acute exacerbations of chronic bronchitis may not allow time for metabolic compensation.
- Blood count—chronic hypoxemia is associated with a bone marrow-mediated increase in hematocrit termed polycythemia; in severe cases, a hematocrit greater than 50% may be encountered.

Emphysema is a pathologic and histologic change in the structure and function of the lung parenchyma. It denotes abnormal and irreversible enlargement of the airspaces distal to the terminal bronchioles. This is accompanied by destruction of their walls without obvious fibrosis. Compared to chronic bronchitis, the pathologic defect is not in the airways but rather in the respiratory unit walls where the loss of elastic tissue results in a loss of appropriate recoil necessary to support expiration.

The clinical appearance of emphysema is noninflammatory in nature and is characterized by shortness of breath, worsening nonreversible airway obstruction, and impaired gas exchange—typically exacerbated by activity:

- Breath sounds—diminished in intensity, reflecting the decreased airflow, prolonged expiratory time, and prominent lung hyperinflation. Other adventitious breath sounds (wheezes, crackles, and rhonchi) are unusual in the absence of concurrent illnesses such as pneumonia.
- Tachycardia—similar to chronic bronchitis, emphysema can present with tachycardia especially with exacerbations or hypoxemia. Pulmonary hypertension is a common secondary finding.
- Imaging—hyperinflation is common with flattening of the hemidiaphragms and an increased anteroposterior chest diameter (Fig. 13.2). The parenchymal destruction associated with emphysema produces enhanced lung peripheral vascular markings often with proximal pulmonary artery dilation.
- Blood gases—the alveolar wall destruction at the capillary level creates an area of high ventilation relative to perfusion (dead space). Most often these patients will compensate to high V/Q ratios by increasing their minute ventilation through increased tidal volume, maintaining nearly normal PO_2 and PCO_2 through most of the disease progression. As in chronic bronchitis, respiratory acidosis and a compensatory metabolic alkalosis are not uncommon in severe emphysema.

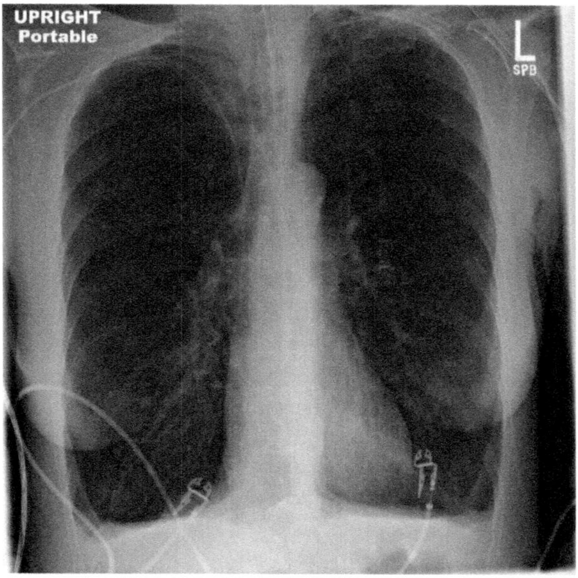

Fig. 13.2 A chest radiograph with the typical findings of COPD. The patient has flattened diaphragms with a narrow mediastinum, indicating air-trapping and hyperinflation

Physiologic Changes in COPD

Supplemental oxygen is given in an attempt to correct a patient's hypoxia to their baseline level of oxygen saturation. This can be delivered by several means, escalating in invasiveness, starting with a simple low-flow nasal cannula through noninvasive positive pressure to invasive mechanical ventilation.

Patients with COPD often have baseline impaired oxygenation due to the loss of alveolar surface areas, increased dead space, and poor respiratory mechanics [1]. Expiratory airflow limitation is a major physiologic alteration in COPD, leading to poor mechanics. Patients attempt to compensate by increasing the inspiratory flow, but the high lung volumes from trapped air make this difficult. Due to the inspiratory compensation and high respiratory drive, patients may develop acute respiratory failure requiring more aggressive support [2].

Noninvasive Ventilation in the COPD Patient

Noninvasive positive-pressure ventilation (NPPV) can be a valuable tool in the acute exacerbation of COPD patients. Its usage during acute exacerbations has been shown to decrease need for mechanical ventilation, overall morbidity, and mortality. Recall that the role of NPPV in respiratory failure is appropriate for those patients who are able to protect their airway and have a condition that, with medical and respiratory support, will resolve relatively quickly. In this patient population, noninvasive continuous positive airway pressure (CPAP) relieves the air-trapping leading to autoPEEP and increased work of breathing. It also functions to keep the soft tissues of the upper airway and oropharynx from collapsing before the onset of inspiration—allowing better triggering of the ventilator by the patient. In many instances, bi-level support, (BiPAP) with inspiratory support, will be appropriate in COPD (Fig. 13.3).

BiPAP may allow for better ventilation and CO_2 clearance than CPAP through augmentation of inspiratory tidal flow and pressures (see Chap. 6). It should be noted that NPPV in any COPD patients may cause dynamic hyperinflation and must be monitored accordingly. In BiPAP, the patient receives a baseline pressure, the expiratory positive airway pressure (EPAP), which is equivalent to PEEP or CPAP. The patient triggers every breath and then receives additional pressure, the inspiratory positive airway pressure (IPAP) (Fig. 13.4).

After the initiation of BiPAP, it is paramount to monitor the therapy for improvement. If patients work of breathing or hypercapnia does not improve, evaluate the tidal volume and inspiratory support flow and pressure. If possible, it is reasonable to attempt to increase the tidal volume via increases in the inspiratory support (IPAP) or inspiratory flow rate. If hypoxemia persists, maneuvers may include increasing the fraction of inspired oxygen (FiO_2) or CPAP/EPAP while also evaluating for signs of autoPEEP.

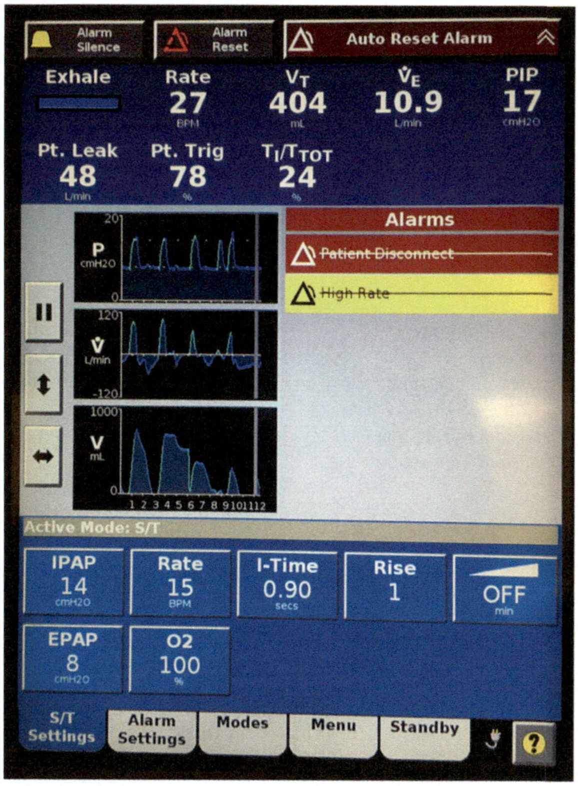

Fig. 13.3 A screen demonstrating the BiPAP settings of a patient with COPD. The IPAP is 14, with an EPAP of 8. Unlike invasive ventilation, where the stated pressure over the PEEP is additive to the peak inspiratory pressure (PIP), by convention in NPPV, the IPAP is the total pressure. The equivalent of the driving pressure in this scenario is 6 mcH_2O

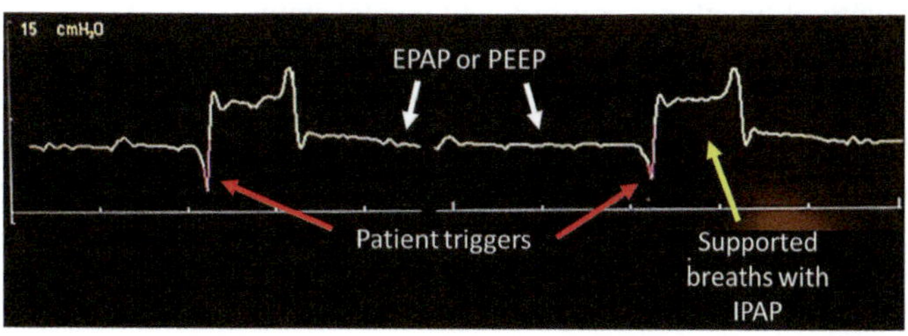

Fig. 13.4 The EPAP is the baseline pressure, and the negative deflections indicate that the patient has triggered the supported breath up to the IPAP. The upward deflection at the end of the breath is likely due to the patient starting an active exhalation process

Spontaneously breathing COPD patients often have active exhalation, even on NPPV. The patient's accessory muscles can start to initiate active exhalation prior to the ventilator cycling to exhalation. This produces an overshoot above the peak inspiratory pressure, as seen in Fig. 13.3. To correct this, adjust the ventilator's end-expiration trigger (if equipped) to better match the patient's inspiratory pattern (Table 13.1) .

Table 13.1 *Initial* settings for NPPV

Setting	Values
Mode	Pressure support mode or BiPAP
Pressures	IPAP or PIP 10 cm H_2O (5 above EPAP) EPAP 5 cm H_2O <8 cm/4 cm (IPAP/EPAP) not advised as it may not be sufficient
Volume	Adjust IPAP targeting a tidal volume of 5–7 mL/kg

Table 13.2 Monitoring and management of NPPV in COPD

Issue	Management
Persistent high work of breathing	Assess mask fit, minute ventilation to ensure adequate ventilation
Altered mental status	Check oxygenation and ventilation to assess for hypoxemia or hypercapnia
Persistent hypercapnia	Increase IPAP by 2 cmH_2O
Persistent hypoxemia	Check tidal volume If less than 8 mL/kg, increase IPAP and EPAP by 2 cmH_2O
Consider pressure limits	IPAP limited to 20–25 cmH_2O to avoid gastric distension EPAP limited to 10–15 cmH_2O
Adjust FiO_2	Use FiO_2 lowest level with an acceptable pulse oximetry reading
Safety measures	Backup apnea respiratory rate 12–16

NPPV has a high rate of success in patients with acute exacerbations of COPD. After initiation and titration of NPPV, many patients show dramatic improvement. After 1–2 h after NPPV initiation, a decrease in $PaCO_2$ (~8 mmHg), improvement of acidosis with (pH > 0.06), and correction of respiratory acidosis are signs of success. Most importantly, however, is assessing the patient clinically for improved work of breathing, comfort, and mental status (Table 13.2).

An unsuccessful trial of NPPV and a need for invasive mechanical ventilation would show any of the following: continued acidosis with a pH < 7.25, hypercapnia >80 mmHg, and decreased mental status suggesting an inability to protect one's airway, respiratory arrest, agitation requiring sedation, hemodynamic instability, bradycardia, or persistent, significant work of breathing. Figure 13.5 shows the BiPAP screen of a patient who is not being well-served by BiPAP and needs to be intubated.

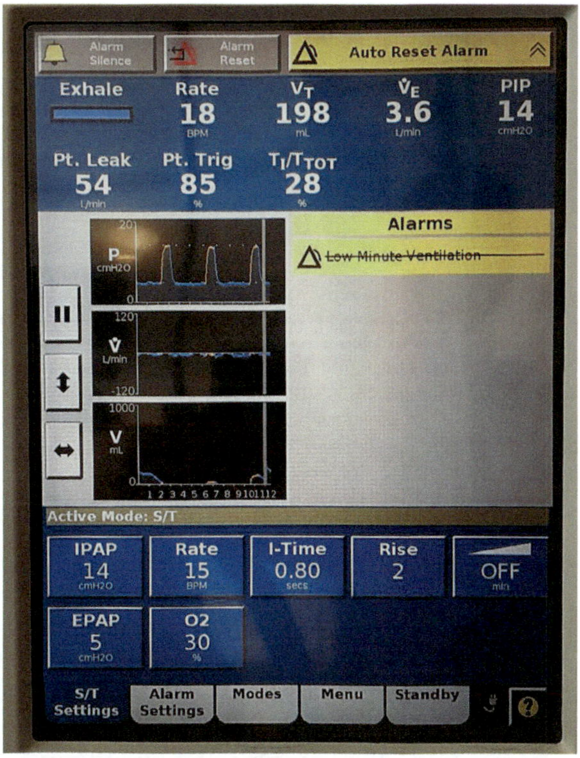

Fig. 13.5 In this scenario, the patient on BiPAP is receiving very tiny tidal volumes with low-minute ventilation. This is clearly ineffective ventilation despite a reasonable IPAP of 14 cmH_2O. This patient should be intubated to ensure adequate ventilation

Intubating the COPD Patient

As with any intubation, preparation is key. Patients with COPD exacerbations exhibit little respiratory reserve, and thus every effort must be made to optimize first look, first pass success utilizing a pre-procedure timeout and utilization of checklist. These patients should be intubated based on the severity of respiratory distress, typically followed by at least 24 h of ventilator support to rest the respiratory muscles.

Full rapid sequence intubation is suggested and includes neuromuscular blockade. Prior to induction, fluid status should be optimized to prevent a possible hemodynamic compromise due to the increased dynamic hyperinflation and intrinsic PEEP. If a patient becomes hypotensive post-induction and is not fluid-responsive, consider an obstructive positive-pressure intrathoracic physiology and disconnect from the ventilator. If there is improvement, consider giving a manual squeeze to the chest, which could reduce the hyperinflation.

Once intubated, the airflow obstruction, low elastic recoil of the lungs, high ventilatory demand, and short expiratory time may lead to air-trapping [2]. This may result in dynamic hyperinflation and auto-positive end-expiratory pressure (autoPEEP) on intrinsic PEEP (iPEEP). As described in Chap. 3, autoPEEP increases intrathoracic pressure. This increased pressure can make triggering difficult in spontaneous ventilator modes, as the patient must overcome the pressure of the

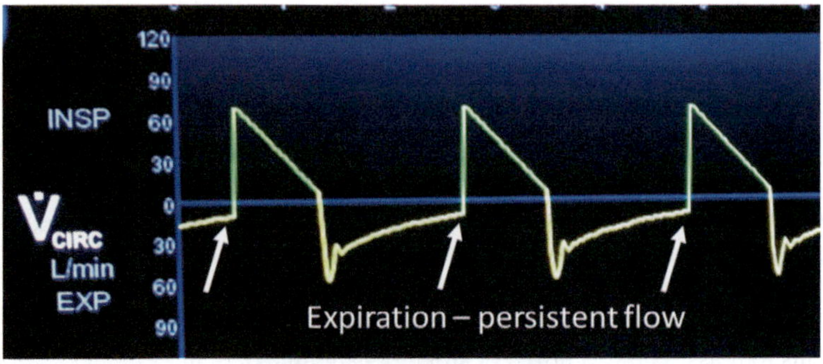

Fig. 13.6 In this image, the flow does not return to the baseline before the next breath is given, indicating that the patient is still exhaling when being forced to inhale. This creates air-trapping. Note that the flow waveform cannot determine the quantity of air-trapping; this is qualitative data only

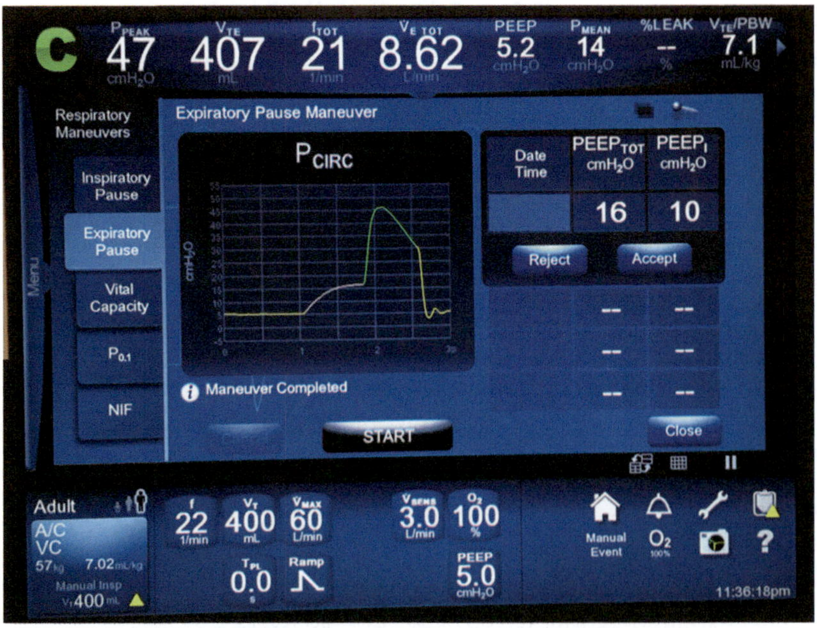

Fig. 13.7 The amount of air-trapping can be quantified by an expiratory hold. In this figure, the PEEP is 10 cmH_2O. The total PEEP is 16 cmH_2O, and the autoPEEP, or intrinsic PEEP, is therefore 6 cmH_2O

autoPEEP to initiate a breath. High levels of autoPEEP may result in hemodynamic consequences as well, as the increased intrathoracic pressure impedes venous return and thus preload. AutoPEEP/dynamic hyperinflation/air-trapping can be diagnosed in several ways and requires astute and frequent reevaluation:

1. Through the slow filling of the manual ventilator bag.
2. The capnography tracing does not reach a plateau.
3. The expiratory flow not reaching zero (Fig. 13.6).
4. Direct measure measurement of the intrinsic PEEP/autoPEEP (Fig. 13.7).

AutoPEEP is measured in patients *without active respiratory effort* using an end-expiratory hold maneuver on the ventilator. The autoPEEP is then calculated by subtracting the external PEEP from the total PEEP.

Ventilator Strategies for the COPD Patient

Targets for ventilation in the COPD patient should be adjusted based on the degree of dynamic hyperinflation and autoPEEP as well as the pH, not the $PaCO_2$. Three factors determine autoPEEP: minute ventilation, I:E ratio, and expiratory time. Minute ventilation is the most important factor; therefore, it targets a smaller tidal volume (Vt) and a slow respiratory rate. Paradoxically, as with asthma (see Chap. 12), allowing time to exhale can improve the ventilation far more than using a higher minute ventilation, as one would do in a patient without obstructive disease. The ultimate goal should be slowly improving the pH, not necessarily fully correcting the $PaCO_2$.

Tools for managing dynamic hyperinflation and autoPEEP are those interventions that allow for more time for exhalation and reduction in breath stacking, such as reducing the respiratory rate or I:E ratio (typically 1:3–1:5). Decreasing the respiratory rate is one the most efficient ways to allow sufficient time to exhale (see Chaps. 3, 7, and 12) [1]. A respiratory rate of 20 only allows for 3 s per respiratory cycle, whereas a respiratory rate of 10 allows 6 s. If both have an inspiratory time of 1 s, the rate of 10 gives 5 s for expiration compared to 2 s for a rate of 20.

Other means of adjusting the ratio of inspiratory time to expiratory time (I:E) ratio are setting it directly on the ventilator, changing the inspiratory time, or adjusting the inspiratory flow rate (Tables 13.3 and 13.4).

Table 13.3 Initial ventilator settings in COPD

Setting	Value
Mode	Assist control
Tidal volume	6–8 mL/kg PBW
Respiratory rate	12–14 bpm; adjust to allow full expiration
Management of I:E ratio	High inspiratory flow 80–100 L/min Short I-time (< 1 s) Set I:E directly (1:3–1:5)
PEEP	5; adjust higher if significant autoPEEP not treated by lowering RR
PIP/Pplat	PIP may be very high with high inspir flows Pplat should be <30 cmH_2O
Trigger	Use flow trigger

Table 13.4 Ventilator settings in the spontaneously breathing patient

Setting	Value
Mode	Pressure support
Tidal volume	PS to generate 6–8 mL/kg
Respiratory rate	Monitor for tachypnea, increased work of breathing
Expiratory sensitivity	Usually set higher than standard 25% (may try 30–35% and increase as needed for synchrony and comfort)
PEEP	5; adjust higher if significant autoPEEP not treated by lowering RR
Trigger	Use minimal flow trigger

References

1. Ward NS, Dushay KM. Clinical concise review: mechanical ventilation of patients with chronic obstructive pulmonary disease. Crit Care Med. 2008;36(5):1614–9. https://doi.org/10.1097/CCM.0B013E318170F0F3.
2. Ahmed SM, Athar M. Mechanical ventilation in patients with chronic obstructive pulmonary disease and bronchial asthma. Indian J Anaesth. 2015;59(9):589. https://doi.org/10.4103/0019-5049.165856.

Trauma

14

Vahé Ender

Introduction

The trauma patient poses unique challenges in care, where therapies usually beneficial in most patients must be weighed for possible harm toward an injured patient. Even if ventilation is needed, the untoward effects of positive pressure ventilation can tip a tenuous bleeding patient into hemodynamic collapse. At a cellular level, mechanical ventilation can potentially trigger an inflammatory response, exacerbating already high levels of inflammation.

While trauma is a diverse, heterogeneous disease, this chapter will aim to provide a pragmatic, evidence-based approach to the mechanical ventilation of these patients, addressing both the acute and long-term phases of the disease.

Considerations for Initiation of Ventilation in the Injured Patient

The decision to initiate mechanical ventilation in a trauma patient is at times controversial. There is little expert medical consensus on whether patients should even be intubated and placed on mechanical ventilation until brought to an operating room for surgical management. These debates may seem academic to a prehospital team providing roadside care to a hypoxic bleeding patient. However, in the sickest trauma patients with an absolute need to correct life-threatening ventilation or oxygenation issues, physiology must be considered, and care should be tailored accordingly.

The risks of mechanical ventilation in the bleeding patient may stem from tenuous hemodynamics, often worsened by the procedures necessary to institute

V. Ender (✉)
Boston MedFlight, Bedford, MA, USA
e-mail: vahe.ender@bostonmedflight.org

© The Author(s), under exclusive license to Springer Nature Switzerland AG 2024

S. R. Wilcox et al. (eds.), *Mechanical Ventilation in Critical Care Transport*,
https://doi.org/10.1007/978-3-031-66782-4_14

mechanical ventilation—from induction and neuromuscular blockade, intubation, and the initiation of positive pressure ventilation. The loss of circulating blood volume from hemorrhage results in decreased vascular pressures, exerting a disproportionate toll on the already low pressures of the venous network, containing 70% of circulating blood volume [1]. Most importantly, this low-pressure vascular system, with a mean pressure of only about 5 mmHg, is subject to compression by external forces [2].

Physiologic breathing resulting from the downward draw of the diaphragm, paired with the outward expansion of the chest wall, generates a *negative* intrathoracic pressure of approximately -6 mmHg. Following the initiation of artificial or assisted ventilation, the thoracic cavity is subjected to a rapid transition to a positive pressure within the chest, potentially impeding the venous flow to the heart.

Considering that venous collapse with positive pressure ventilation can be seen *in a volume-replete patient*, it is easy to imagine this collapse being far worse in hemorrhagic shock. The resulting drop in venous return decreases right atrial filling, affecting left ventricular output to the body. In response to low perfusion, sympathetic activation will result in vasoconstriction and shunting of blood to restore venous systemic pressures. This sympathetic stimulus also influences cardiac function, increasing contractility, stroke volume, and heart rate. These effects are part of the body's attempts to restore essential organ perfusion.

The use of induction agents will blunt the catecholaminergic response to hemorrhage. While the use of ketamine or etomidate has shown a lower incidence of hypotension over other agents, all induction agents do have the potential for negative hemodynamic effects. No evidence currently shows any benefit to reducing dosing of these agents though in general, reduced dosing is felt to be reasonable in hemodynamically unstable patients.

The decision to intubate a patient is complex, and no protocolized, universal approach is possible. The risk of harm must be weighed against the benefits of the intervention. With the risk of cardiovascular collapse, intubation should be reserved for patients with clear hypoventilation, hypoxia, or aspiration not correctible by other means (Fig. 14.1). A bleeding patient with a depressed mental status but with adequate ventilation and oxygenation may benefit from deferred intubation to allow for earlier operative hemostasis. When the team does decide to intubate, it is important to mitigate harm by ensuring a well-equipped, high-performing team is available to provide the safest intubation: a team providing high rates of first-pass success providing careful medication management. When intubation is deemed necessary, it should be done in conjunction with the correction of life threats at the same time and supported by the use of blood products and, in some cases, IV push vasopressors.

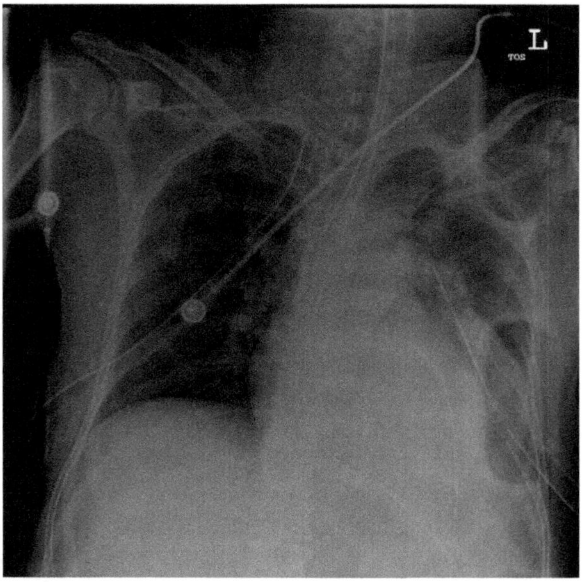

Fig. 14.1 Chest X-ray demonstrating a traumatic diaphragmatic rupture. This image highlights some of the profound heterogeneity and physiologic complexity that can be seen in trauma patients

Considerations for the Ventilatory Management of the Injured Patient

Unfortunately, there is limited human research available to guide the best ventilatory strategy for unstable trauma patients. Some texts have taken the position to decrease the frequency of compressing the patient's vasculature by positive pressure ventilation. More based on theory than evidence, this approach proposes a low-pressure, low respiratory rate strategy with no baseline PEEP. This approach risks hypoventilation, and atelectotrauma, as well as the potential to increase right ventricular workload due to collapsed alveolar vasculature—potentially resulting in worsened metabolic and hemodynamic derangement.

A pragmatic approach is to focus on providing the lowest pressures necessary for adequate ventilation and oxygenation while also providing just enough minute ventilation to prevent worsening acidosis.

The necessary volume to ventilate effectively is patient-dependent and can be assessed by the bedside evaluation of chest rise and lung sounds. Tidal volumes of 5–7 mL/kg PBW are a reasonable starting point. Following assurance of effective ventilation, the associated peak inspiratory pressures (PIPs) should be evaluated to mitigate barotrauma risk. A starting respiratory rate should be higher to account for the increased metabolic needs of a patient in shock (see Chap. 10), but deliberate hyperventilation with large tidal volumes should be avoided, as animal models have shown increased mortality likely due to the resulting increase in venous compression [3]. While some debate exists regarding the definition of "physiologic" positive end-expiratory pressure (PEEP), a reasonable value of 5 cmH_2O provides adequate airway stenting to avoid atelectotrauma.

Some specific patient injuries result in some significant implications worth discussing in greater detail.

Brain Injury

Following injury to the brain, efforts must be focused on preventing secondary injury (see Chap. 15). Hypoxia has been found to be independently associated with worsened outcomes following traumatic brain injury, cutting survival by up to 28.1% [4]. This mortality increase surpassed the effects of hypotension, indicating the importance of protecting the injured patient from desaturation. Interestingly, this trend toward decreased survival is also seen with extreme hyperoxia ($paO_2 > 500$ mmHg) due to an increased production of reactive oxidative species resulting in brain tissue injury [5]. As such, a goal saturation of 93–95% provides reasonable guardrails against risk associated with the extremes of oxygen therapy.

Carbon dioxide helps regulate cerebral perfusion. Decreased CO_2 levels can induce vasoconstriction, historically used to decrease cerebral volume. Unfortunately, this can result in cerebral hypoperfusion, worsening perfusion in regions of the injured brain already threatened by edema leading to worsened ischemia. As such, routine hyperventilation is not recommended and should only be used as a last resort for refractory cases. Instead, simple maneuvers such as elevation of the head, loosening cervical collars, adequate sedation and analgesia, and hyperosmolar therapy may yield a greater benefit with less risk for harm.

Airway Injury

Injuries can occur all the way down the conducting airway from the trachea distally to the lung itself. The decision to intubate is challenging, as the patient may sometimes be able to protect their own airway, and intubation can potentially lead to manual airway disruption. Conversely, the window to intubate may be transient before the swelling and bleeding preclude the ability to capture the airway. Defects in the trachea and its branches result in significant challenges due to potential difficulties with ventilation and the accumulation of mediastinal and subcutaneous air. Without an injury where the advancement of an endotracheal tube may isolate ventilation distal to the defect or the opportunity for the placement of a chest tube, the goal should be minimizing PIPs to the lowest pressure necessary to provide observable chest rise. Temporary hypoventilation may be considered for prehospital care until temporary or definitive surgical management can be accessed.

Pneumothorax

The ventilatory management of patients with thoracic trauma resulting in pneumothorax has long been debated. Without a chest drain in place, tidal breaths may convert a simple pneumothorax to tension pneumothorax as increasing amounts of air accumulate in the pleural space. Not all pneumothoraces subject to PPV will worsen, with some guidelines recommending small pneumothoraces (10–15%) be subject to a "watch and wait" approach over the empiric placement of a chest drain [6]. A reasonable approach is that a clinically apparent pneumothorax (dyspnea, hypoxia) in a spontaneously breathing patient likely requires placement of a thoracostomy tube prior to or immediately following of PPV to prevent tension physiology. In patients with radiographically evident pneumothorax who appear clinically well, it may be reasonable to monitor the patient instead, while keeping a low threshold for intervention (Table 14.1).

Pulmonary Injury

Patients who suffer thoracic trauma often develop an underappreciated injury: pulmonary contusion. This injury is surprisingly common—seen in 17–75% of blunt trauma patients. It also presents with a broad spectrum of severity—from occult contusion only detected on CT imaging to diffuse life-threatening injury causing respiratory failure [7]. The ventilatory approach is dependent on the severity of the presentation. A patient with significant blunt thoracic trauma may develop diffuse bilateral disease consistent with acute respiratory distress syndrome (ARDS) (see Chap. 11). These patients require a similar approach, with careful titration of ventilation to target functional lung through driving pressure measurements and optimization of oxygenation through best PEEP evaluations. Depending upon the

Table 14.1 Key management strategies for suspected/confirmed injury patterns

Injury	Management
Hemorrhagic shock	Strongly consider risks of intubation/ventilation—Possible hemodynamic collapse If possible, optimize with blood, vasopressors prior to ventilation Use low TV, low PEEP (5 cmH_2O), RR to address metabolic acidosis
Traumatic brain injury	Target normal values—Normal pCO_2, normal PaO_2 Use low-moderate PEEP to support oxygenation
Airway injury	Decision to intubate very challenging Avoiding worsening injury in the field can be impossible (best done in hospital with fiberoptics) If able to bypass injury, may need to ventilate one lung Patients may need chest drainage for pneumothorax Keep pressures low
Pulmonary injury/lung contusion	Varied presentation from mild to severe ARDS Low TV, higher RR, higher PEEP If unilateral, can try good lung down

distribution of injury in trauma, patients may present with severe unilateral disease leaving one remaining functional lung. In these patients, placement of the "good lung down" may leverage additional blood flow being provided to the uninjured lung, improving oxygenation, but one must be cautious against soiling of the good lung should there be active bleeding into the injured lung.

Finally, considering the high vascularity of the lung and it being prone to developing dysfunction in systemic illness, it is important to consider trauma as a common cause of ARDS. This pathology, and its most optimal approach, is covered in Chap. 11 in greater detail.

The Role of the Transport Team in the Care of the Injured Patient

Helicopter Emergency Medical Services (HEMS) and Critical Care Transport (CCT) teams represent a broad spectrum of care including providing advanced interventions at point-of-injury to performing complex secondary transfer of critically injured patients requiring tertiary-or quaternary-level care. The breadth of work is reflected in not only the pathology encountered but in approaches to care.

Patients in the prehospital environment present with an early manifestation of disease that may be undetectable, only to bloom later during their inpatient admission. The complexity and goals of prehospital intervention also differ from that of a complex trauma transfer.

The initial goals of prehospital intervention focus on providing fundamental lifesaving care while avoiding secondary injury resulting from hypoxia or hypotension. The benefit of interventions should always be weighed against the potential harms due to resulting delays in transport from procedures and diagnostic capabilities.

The limited diagnostic capabilities in the field contrast with the care of the secondary trauma transfer. While a transfer patient can be of low complexity, such as a patient transferred from one center to another for an emergency surgery, many can suffer from complex problems affecting multiple organs requiring "precision medicine" while managing a broad range of clinical problems. This dichotomy requires CCT/HEMS clinicians to be highly versatile providers who are able to titrate their care based on patient need while being cognizant that trauma is a time-sensitive disease.

References

1. Rothe CF. Reflex control of veins and vascular capacitance. Physiol Rev. 1983;63:1281–342.
2. Shah P, Louis MA. Physiology, Central Venous Pressure. StatPearls Publishing; 2024.
3. Aufderheide TP, Sigurdsson G, Pirrallo RG, Yannopoulos D, McKnite S, von Briesen C, et al. Hyperventilation-induced hypotension during cardiopulmonary resuscitation. Circulation. 2004;109:1960–5.
4. Spaite DW, Hu C, Bobrow BJ, Chikani V, Barnhart B, Gaither JB, Denninghoff KR, Adelson PD, Keim SM, Viscusi C, Mullins T, Sherrill D. The effect of combined out-of-hospital hypotension and hypoxia on mortality in major traumatic brain injury. Ann Emerg Med. 2017;53:443.

5. Davis DP, Meade W, Sise MJ, Kennedy F, Simon F, Tominaga G, Steele J, Coimbra R. Both hypoxemia and extreme hyperoxemia may be detrimental in patients with severe traumatic brain injury. J Neurotrauma. 2009;26(12):2217–23.
6. de Moya M, Brasel KJ, Brown CVR, et al. Evaluation and management of traumatic pneumothorax: a Western trauma association critical decisions algorithm. J Trauma Acute Care Surg. 2022;92(1):103–7.
7. Simon B, Ebert J, Bokhari F, Capella J, Emhoff T, Hayward T 3rd, Rodriguez A, Smith L. Management of pulmonary contusion and flail chest: an eastern Association for the Surgery of trauma practice management guideline. Eastern Association for the Surgery of Trauma. J Trauma Acute Care Surg. 2012;73:S351.

Neuro Critical Care

15

Cayleigh Montano

Neurologic injuries that require mechanical ventilation represent some of the most severe emergencies seen by practicing clinicians. The primary injury to the brain, whether it be from traumatic brain injury, intracerebral hemorrhage, ischemic stroke, or seizures, is irreversible; however, an informed approach to resuscitation that emphasizes oxygenation, ventilation, and hemodynamic goals can benefit the patient and prevent secondary brain injury.

Mechanical ventilation can alter oxygen and carbon dioxide compositions in the brain. Oxygen is vital for neuronal survival [1]. There are two requirements to maintain oxygen in the brain: cerebral blood flow and adequate arterial oxygen content. Optimizing mechanical ventilation can optimize cerebral oxygenation. Still, ventilation plays a vital role. Hypercapnia results in cerebral vasodilation, increasing cerebral blood flow and intracranial pressures. Conversely, hypocapnia causes cerebral vasoconstriction, reducing cerebral blood flow and perfusion and decreasing intracranial pressure (Fig. 15.1). Preventing hypercapnia and hypocapnia, except in the acutely herniating patient, protects the brain from secondary injury.

C. Montano (✉)
Boston MedFlight, Bedford, MA, USA
e-mail: cayleigh.montano@bostonmedflight.org

© The Author(s), under exclusive license to Springer Nature Switzerland AG 2024

S. R. Wilcox et al. (eds.), *Mechanical Ventilation in Critical Care Transport*,
https://doi.org/10.1007/978-3-031-66782-4_15

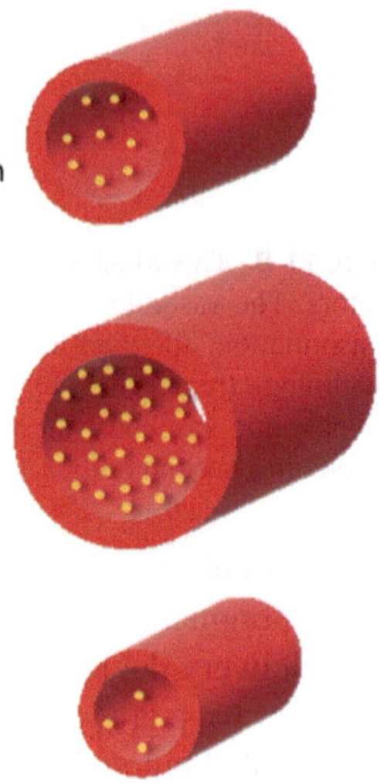

Fig. 15.1 Demonstration of the vasodilation and vasoconstriction seen with changes in the pCO_2. This vascular reactivity mandates close management of ventilation in patients with neurologic injury

Traumatic Brain Injury

In 2020–2021, the CDC estimated 214,110 traumatic brain injury (TBI)-related hospitalizations and 69,473 related deaths [1]. Prehospital guidelines from The Brain Trauma Foundation recommend establishing a secure airway "by the most appropriate means available" for patients with a Glasgow Coma Scale <9, an inability to protect their airway, or $SpO_2 < 90\%$ that does not respond to supplemental oxygen [2]. Research has shown that rapid sequence intubation establishes the best opportunity for first-pass success [3]. While important for all patients, first-pass success is especially important in TBI as it has less risk for hypoxemia, hypercarbia, and stimulus induced elevation in intracranial pressure (ICP) than subsequent attempts. Preventing hypoxemia is important in all steps, including the need for thorough preoxygenation and attention to oxygenation and ventilation via bag-valve mask before placing the patient on a ventilator. However, after intubation, it is crucial to prevent unintentional hypoxemia, hypercapnia, and hypocapnia. Special considerations for cervical restrictions should be considered, and tools that limit cervical manipulation, such as video laryngoscopy and the gum elastic bougie, should be available at the bedside.

Both hypoxemia and hyperoxia are associated with increased mortality and poor outcomes among TBI patients [4]. Therefore, the goal of oxygenation for TBI patients should be SpO_2 94–99% and partial pressure of oxygen in arterial blood (PaO_2) 80–120 mmHg [5].

The effects of positive end-expiratory pressure (PEEP) on intracranial pressures are not well researched and remain controversial. Several studies have shown that PEEP does not affect intracranial pressures (ICP), yet others show that PEEP >12 cmH_2O negatively impacts ICP [6–8]. For the hypoxic patient requiring PEEP to achieve satisfactory oxygenation, the clinician must assess the benefits of PEEP while simultaneously supporting the patient's hemodynamic status, thus ensuring a physiological cerebral perfusion pressure. Intracranial pressure monitors can be used to guide the titration of PEEP in patients with acute respiratory distress syndrome (ARDS) and acute brain injury.

Hypoventilation leads to hypercapnia and should be avoided. Hypercapnia can result in cerebral vasodilation, thereby increasing blood flow and intracranial pressures (Fig. 15.1). Clinicians should avoid further increasing ICP in patients with presumed or known elevated ICP.

Quantitative capnometry via end-tidal carbon dioxide monitoring ($EtCO_2$) is a valuable tool for airway safety but reflects arterial pCO_2 and minute ventilation only in a steady-state physiology condition that is uncommonly achieved in a critical care patient or in transport. (Please see Chap. 5 for more details.) Empirical estimates and physical assessments of physiologically appropriate ventilation must be confirmed with blood gas, once one is available.

Hyperventilation should also be avoided unless the patient presents with clinical signs of imminent acute herniation (e.g., loss of brainstem reflexes, irregular or absent respiratory patterns, profound hypertension, bradycardia, and coma). Clinicians should only consider hyperventilation as a last resort to bridge the patient to emergent neurosurgery. Osmotic therapy and mean arterial pressure (MAP) augmentation should be implemented well before hyperventilation [9]. Hypocapnia will result in cerebral vasoconstriction, reducing cerebral blood flow and perfusion and decreasing intracranial pressure at the expense of blood flow to injured areas of the brain [10]. Hyperventilation should only be used while evaluating or transporting to a facility for lifesaving interventions such as the placement of an external ventricular drain, decompressive craniectomy, or abdominal decompression.

Sometimes, the most straightforward interventions yield the best results. Clinicians should ensure that TBI patients are adequately sedated and minimally stimulated while they recover. Elevating the head of the patient's bed and loosening restrictive collars to maximize cephalic venous return may significantly decrease intracranial pressures.

Spontaneous Intracerebral Hemorrhage

Spontaneous intracerebral hemorrhage (ICH) is defined as nontraumatic bleeding into the brain parenchyma. Ventilatory strategies for patients with ICH are similar to those for patients with TBIs. Early management should focus on airway, breathing, and circulation; detailed neurologic assessment; and a high suspicion for deterioration due to early hematoma expansion or acute hydrocephalus [11]. Preventing hypoxia through adequate ventilation and oxygenation will mitigate secondary brain injury.

Special considerations for hemostatic therapy, blood pressure control, and surgical management play a role in improving outcomes [12]. As with patients who have a traumatic brain injury, hypoxemia and hyperoxemia should be avoided in

ICH. Normocapnia should be achieved with reservation of hyperventilation in patients with acute herniation while waiting for emergent definitive treatment.

Ischemic Stroke

Every year, more than 795,000 people in the United States suffer from stroke, and about 87% of all strokes are ischemic strokes [13]. Ischemic stroke patients can be treated with medications such as alteplase and tenecteplase or with endovascular clot retrieval. The focus of Critical Care Transport clinicians is on preventing secondary injury while awaiting definitive treatment. It is critical to be mindful of patients with large hemispheric strokes who may develop malignant edema and/or hemorrhagic transformation.

Stroke patients may require intubation when they are unable to protect their airway. Ischemic stroke patients may have preserved consciousness but may not be able to manage their secretions. Oropharyngeal dysfunction puts them at high risk for aspiration and further respiratory compromise [14]. Key ventilator management, like those of most patients with acute brain injury, should focus on preventing hypoxia and hyperoxemia [15] while maintaining normocapnia unless they are acutely herniating.

Status Epilepticus

Status epilepticus is defined as a seizure lasting longer than 5 min or when the patient has more than one seizure without returning to their baseline mentation between seizures. These patients are at increased risk of hypoxia, aspiration, and respiratory compromise. Patients who are in status epilepticus will likely require higher doses of antiepileptics, often further complicating their ability to protect their airway and breathing adequately. Intubation should focus on the overall clinical course to prevent hypoxia and worsening acidosis that can be associated with prolonged periods of seizures [16]. Intubation may allow for more aggressive treatment with medications such as propofol. These medications may halt seizures, reducing the risk of refractory status epilepticus and supra-refractory status epilepticus. Once intubated, the minute ventilation should be titrated to their acid-base status.

References

1. Centers for Disease Control and Prevention. 2023. Tbi data. https://www.cdc.gov/traumatic-braininjury/data/index.html.
2. Marehbian J, Muehlschlegel S, Edlow BL, Hinson HE, Hwang DY. Medical management of the severe traumatic brain injury patient. Neurocrit Care. 2017;27(3):430–46. https://doi.org/10.1007/s12028-017-0408-5.

3. Okubo M, Gibo K, Hagiwara Y, Nakayama Y, Hasegawa K. The effectiveness of rapid sequence intubation (rsi) versus non-rsi in emergency department: an analysis of multicenter prospective observational study. Int J Emerg Med. 2017;10(1):1. https://doi.org/10.1186/s12245-017-0129-8.
4. Davis DP, Meade W, Sise MJ, Kennedy F, Simon F, Tominaga G, Steele J, Coimbra R. Both hypoxemia and extreme hyperoxemia may be detrimental in patients with severe traumatic brain injury. J Neurotrauma. 2009;26(12):2217–23. https://doi.org/10.1089/neu.2009.0940.
5. Robba C, Poole D, McNett M, Asehnoune K, Bösel J, Bruder N, Chieregato A, Cinotti R, Duranteau J, Einav S, Ercole A, Ferguson N, Guerin C, Siempos II, Kurtz P, Juffermans NP, Mancebo J, Mascia L, McCredie V, Stevens RD. Mechanical ventilation in patients with acute brain injury: recommendations of the european society of intensive care medicine consensus. Intensive Care Med. 2020;46(12):2397–410. https://doi.org/10.1007/s00134-020-06283-0.
6. Kim JA, Wahlster S, LaBuzetta J, Nobleza CS, Johnson NJ, Rubinos C, Malaiyandi D, O'Phelan KH, Mainali S, Sarwal A, Gilmore EJ. Focused management of patients with severe acute brain injury and ards. Chest. 2022;161(1):140–51. https://doi.org/10.1016/j.chest.2021.08.066.
7. Boone MD, Jinadasa SP, Mueller A, Shaefi S, Kasper EM, Hanafy KA, O'Gara BP, Talmor DS. The effect of positive end-expiratory pressure on intracranial pressure and cerebral hemodynamics. Neurocrit Care. 2016;26(2):174–81. https://doi.org/10.1007/s12028-016-0328-9.
8. Robba C, Ball L, Nogas S, Battaglini D, Messina A, Brunetti I, Minetti G, Castellan L, Rocco PM, Pelosi P. Effects of positive end-expiratory pressure on lung recruitment, respiratory mechanics, and intracranial pressure in mechanically ventilated brain-injured patients. Front Physiol. 2021;12:711273. https://doi.org/10.3389/fphys.2021.711273.
9. Godoy D, Seifi A, Garza D, Lubillo-Montenegro S, Murillo-Cabezas F. Hyperventilation therapy for control of posttraumatic intracranial hypertension. Front Neurol. 2017;8:250. https://doi.org/10.3389/fneur.2017.00250.
10. Zhang Z, Guo Q, Wang E. Hyperventilation in neurological patients. Curr Opin Anaesthesiol. 2019;32(5):568–73. https://doi.org/10.1097/aco.0000000000000764.
11. Specogna AV, Turin TC, Patten SB, Hill MD. Factors associated with early deterioration after spontaneous intracerebral hemorrhage: a systematic review and meta-analysis. PLoS One. 2014;9(5):e96743. https://doi.org/10.1371/journal.pone.0096743.
12. de Oliveira Manoel A, Goffi A, Zampieri F, Turkel-Parrella D, Duggal A, Marotta TR, Macdonald R, Abrahamson S. The critical care management of spontaneous intracranial hemorrhage: a contemporary review. Crit Care. 2016;20(1):272. https://doi.org/10.1186/s13054-016-1432-0.
13. Centers for Disease Control and Prevention. 2023. Stroke facts. https://www.cdc.gov/stroke/facts.htm.
14. Bevers MB, Kimberly W. Critical care management of acute ischemic stroke. Curr Treat Options Cardiovasc Med. 2017;19(6):41. https://doi.org/10.1007/s11936-017-0542-6.
15. Vincent J-L, Taccone F, He X. Harmful effects of hyperoxia in postcardiac arrest, sepsis, traumatic brain injury, or stroke: the importance of individualized oxygen therapy in critically ill patients. Can Respir J. 2017;2017:1–7. https://doi.org/10.1155/2017/2834956.
16. Diler Y, Özdemir S, Altunok I, Emre Eroğlu S. Relationship between seizures and metabolic acidosis: a prospective observational study. Front Emerg Med. 2022;6:1. https://doi.org/10.18502/fem.v6i2.8715.

Pediatric Ventilator Management

16

Jamie Eastman

Intubation and mechanical ventilation for pediatric patients are high-risk procedures. Pediatric patients are intubated three to six times less often than adults in the emergency department [1]. While many principles of mechanical ventilation are similar between adult and pediatric patients, there are numerous key differences. Critical care transport clinicians who may care for children should be educated and proficient in managing ventilators for those pediatric patients. The literature on pediatric mechanical ventilation is limited to retrospective and observational studies. Very few, if any, randomized controlled trials exist. Most of the recognized literature in this field is consensus data from leading clinicians [2]. Much of the information is extrapolated from adult mechanical ventilation research and adapted to the pediatric patient.

Pediatric Physiology

The respiratory physiology of children is very different than that of adults. Neonatal physiology is quite different and is addressed in Chap. 17, though there is certainly overlap at the end of the neonatal period (30 days of life). Even non-neonates have differences that must be recognized for good ventilation management, however.

Children tend to have proportionally higher metabolic rates and consume oxygen more rapidly than full grown adults. They also have a lower functional residual capacity in the lungs, making them particularly susceptible to desaturation [3]. For patients encountered prior to intubation, the transport clinicians should recognize impending respiratory failure, focusing on the child's appearance, work of breathing, and skin circulation [4]. Hypoxemia, bradycardia, and altered mental status may be signs of impending respiratory and/or cardiac arrest.

J. Eastman (✉)
Boston MedFlight, Bedford, MA, USA
e-mail: jamie.eastman@bostonmedflight.org

© The Author(s), under exclusive license to Springer Nature Switzerland AG 2024

S. R. Wilcox et al. (eds.), *Mechanical Ventilation in Critical Care Transport*,
https://doi.org/10.1007/978-3-031-66782-4_16

Pediatric patients have smaller, more compliant airways, especially in younger children. The flexible, cartilaginous ribs of young patients are often horizontal, providing poor mechanical advantage for air movement. This means that infants and toddlers are more dependent upon their diaphragms for ventilation [3, 4]. Alveoli grow and develop throughout childhood into adolescence [3], meaning that young children have proportionally less surface area for gas exchange than do older children and adults. It is also important to recognize that lungs develop in proportion to the length/height of the patient, and not girth, such that an obese child will still have the pulmonary physiology of a child and not necessarily that of an equal weight (but taller) adult.

Indications for Intubation and Mechanical Ventilation in Children

The necessity for intubation and mechanical ventilation in the pediatric population mirrors the adult indications. Respiratory failure, worsening respiratory and metabolic acidosis, altered mental status with loss of airway control, airway obstruction, and central nervous system depression are all appropriate indications for intubation and mechanical intubation. Respiratory failure in the pediatric population typically stems from acute respiratory distress syndrome (ARDS), restrictive airway complications such as asthma, or infectious processes such as pneumonia. Worsening acidosis from sepsis, metabolic derangements, and congenital disease are also common. Altered mental status and central nervous system depression from toxic ingestions, glycemic derangements, epilepsy, traumatic or spontaneous neurologic injury, or neurologic malignancy are well possible reasons for the necessity of mechanical ventilation.

Setting the Ventilator in Pediatric Patients

Mode

Selecting the mode of invasive ventilation for the pediatric patient should be in conjunction with an expert in the care of critically ill children, such as via communication with medical direction. It is best practice to share these discussions with sending and receiving multidisciplinary medical teams. There is currently no literature to support the selection of one mode of ventilation over the other in all pediatric cases [5, 6]. The preference for all pediatric patients on the ventilator should be to breathe spontaneously [7]. However, during transport and while in extremis, typically full control of gas exchange is required to resuscitate the patient. Assist Control (AC) offers complete ventilation control, and assist control, pressure cycled (AC/PC, or pressure control) protects from barotrauma while inflating small lungs. There is such wide variation in practice, so it is challenging to state what "conventional" ventilation may be. Despite consensus guidelines [2], a prior survey found that about 75% of pediatric patients were ventilated with a volume control mode [2].

Pressure and Tidal Volume

When selecting the ventilation pressure on a pressure control strategy, the recommended maximum plateau pressure (Pplat) is ≤28 cmH_2O, determined by expert consensus [7]. There are no specific data to support the starting pressure for pediatric patients; however, a peak inspiratory pressure (PIP) of 15–20 cmH_20 is a reasonable initial value [6].

There are fewer studies of tidal volumes in pediatrics than in adult medicine. When setting pressure, the Pediatric Acute Lung Injury Consensus Conference (PALICC) recommends a target tidal volume of 5–8 mL/kg *ideal* body weight [6]. As with adults, clinicians have a predicted adopted body weight (PBW) versus actual body weight, but no pediatric data support this practice [6]. ARDSnet has been adopted in the pediatric population, supporting a 6 mL/kg tidal volume ideal body weight [8] although there is no yet demonstrated clear association between tidal volumes and mortality in pediatrics. Many initial standard tidal volumes begin around 8 mL/kg of PBW [2], and expert consensus recommends avoiding tidal volumes over 10 mL/kg PBW [7].

When caring for a patient on a pressure control mode, to increase the measured tidal volume, incrementally increase the set pressure, or (less commonly) increase the inspiratory time or flow rate. To decrease the measured tidal volume, incrementally decrease the set pressure, inspiratory time, or flow rate. Substantial changes in ventilatory settings should be evaluated with a subsequent blood gas value, and, if appropriate, involve consultation with expert medical direction.

Rate

Respiratory rate selection is based on the desired minute ventilation (Mv = Tidal volume × respiratory rate). Normal minute ventilation for an adult is ~100 mL/kg/min for ideal body weight for a healthy patient. This has been adapted to pediatric patients as well [6]. Patients with acidosis (pH < 7.15) may require higher minute ventilation for gas exchange to promote respiratory compensation. Normal starting respiratory rates typically start at 20–30 breaths per minute for pediatric patients.

PEEP

Physiologic peak end-expiratory pressure (PEEP) for an adult is generally felt to be 5 cmH_2O—consensus criteria also support this level in pediatrics. Some clinicians may choose to increase PEEP, preferentially to increasing oxygen (FiO_2) to decrease the risk for free radicals—assuming there is not overdistension [6]. With some diagnoses such as ARDS and bronchopulmonary dysplasia (BPD), higher PEEP settings may be required [9]. PEEP >10 cmH_2O should involve discussion with medical direction and/or receiving multidisciplinary team before transport. Conversely, in restrictive airways such as asthma, PEEP may be set to less than 5 cmH_2O [9].

FiO_2

Oxygen concentration should be titrated based on available real-time measurement of blood oxygenation. In the vast majority of circumstances, this is the pulse oximeter—however, at times, this may require review of arterial blood gas partial pressure of oxygen (PaO_2). Initial treatment may require 100% FiO_2 during resuscitation, but oxygen should be weaned as appropriate. The risk for complications of oxygen toxicity is greater in children than adults. Many clinicians will initiate FiO_2 at 60% as a safe starting point.

Inspiratory Time

Setting inspiratory time (I-time) is age- and disease-based. Typically, pediatric I-time is 0.5–0.8 s. Older patients may require longer I-times. Table 16.1 highlights some common I-times defined by age. As with adults, shortening I-times may be required for patients with restricted airway diseases such as asthma to allow for longer expiratory time.

Putting all these recommendations together, Table 16.2 provides suggested initial ventilator settings.

Table 16.1 Initial respiratory rate and I-time by age

Age-based settings	Respiratory rate	Inspiratory time
Infant (1 year)	25–30	0.5–0.6
Child (1–5 years)	20–25	0.6–0.8
Child (5–12 years)	15–20	0.6–0.8
Adolescent	12–15	0.8–1.2

Table 16.2 Additional suggested initial settings

Starting ventilator settings	Value
Mode	Assist control
Tidal volume	5–8 mL/kg IBW
PIP	< 28 cmH_2O
PEEP	5 cmH_2O
FiO_2	60–100%

Monitoring Ventilated Pediatric Patients

Continuous monitoring of mechanically ventilated pediatric patients is crucial to avoid adverse events or recognize complications before significant physiologic decline. Clinicians must ensure that they have appropriate equipment designed and sized for pediatric patients, as attempting to fit adult equipment to pediatric patients can lead to diagnostic errors [4]. Changes to mechanical ventilation should be made utilizing near real-time oxygenation monitoring via pulse oximetry, in conjunction with recent (and as appropriate—serial) blood gas monitoring and medical direction. In the absence of recent blood gas review, end-tidal CO_2 ($EtCO_2$) can assist with guiding treatment though it is important to recognize the significant limitations in the absolute value of $EtCO_2$ particularly in patients with shock or depressed cardiac output.

Resistance and Compliance

Monitoring resistance and compliance is crucial in pediatric patients. See Chap. 7 for a detailed discussion of pressures on the ventilator. Resistance is the measure of the flow of air through the airway system. Increases in resistance would indicate constriction of the airway. Compliance is a measure of the stiffness of the lungs or the body outside the respiratory system (chest wall burns, obesity.) Decreases in compliance would indicate pathologies such as consolidation, edema, inflammation, or fibrosis within the lung, and higher pressures are needed for gas exchange.

Monitoring Oxygenation

The 2017 Pediatric Mechanical Ventilation Consensus Conference recommended that the SpO_2 levels in pediatric ARDS should be 92–97% when PEEP is <10 cm H_2O and 88–92% when the PEEP is >10 cm H_2O with the lowest FiO_2 possible [7].

In patients with worsening ARDS, monitoring of the Oxygenation Index ($OI = MAP \times Fio_2 \times 100/Pao_2$) is an effective tool in deciding the next treatments [10], such as the need to escalate to different ventilator modes, inhaled pulmonary vasodilators, or extracorporeal membrane oxygenation. However, calculating an OI may be challenging as arterial blood gases (ABGs) are less commonly checked in pediatrics than they are in adult medicine and may not be easily available [2].

Because of the limitations in ABGs, expert panels have recommended the use of the oxygen saturation index (OSI) as an alternative to quantify hypoxemia in children [6]. The OSI uses data that can be easily obtained in transport, including the FiO_2, the SpO_2, and the mean airway pressure ($\bar{P}aw$).

$$OSI = \left(\frac{\left[Fio_2 \times Paw \times 100 \right]}{Spo_2} \right)$$

Monitoring Ventilation

When able, checking a blood gas to evaluate the pCO_2 of ventilated patient is appropriate. Expert consensus recommends targeting normal CO_2 levels, 35–45 mmHg, in children with previously normal lungs [7]. However, permissive hypercapnia may also be tolerated to allow lung protection, ideally with a pH > 7.20, but there is no specific pH limit. However, in children at risk for pulmonary hypertension, right ventricular dysfunction, or traumatic brain injury, it is recommended to target normal pCO_2 and pH [7].

As with adults, the $ETCO_2$ reflects numerous aspects of physiology, and it cannot be assumed to be an equivalent of the $PaCO_2$. The $ETCO_2$ can be correlated with a blood gas, and trends can be followed. However, the relationship between the pCO_2 and $ETCO_2$ can change with increasing dead space, reduced cardiac output, or suboptimal ventilator management. Of primary importance, though, in continuous quantitative $EtCO_2$ monitoring in all mechanically ventilated patient is early recognition of endotracheal tube malposition or dislodgement in transport—well before oxygenation or hemodynamics suffer.

Adverse Events in Pediatric Patients

As with adult patients, mechanical ventilation poses a risk for both barotrauma and volutrauma. Ensuring that pressures and volumes do not exceed limits is crucial to preventing healthcare induced injury. As mentioned previously, safe Pplat should not exceed 28 cmH_2O, and tidal volumes greater than 10 mL/kg should be avoided [6]. Clinical situations approaching or at these extremes should ideally be managed in conjunction with expert guidance from medical direction experts and experts in pediatric critical care.

Children are at risk for desaturation with movement, as are adults (see Chap. 4.) Pediatric patients are at a significantly elevated risk of endotracheal tube dislodgement with movement, given their differences in anatomy. Minimal inadvertent head flexion or extension has commensurate movement of the endotracheal tube—potentially resulting in main-stem placement or extubation. Particular care must be utilized when moving a mechanically ventilated child, often mandating a dedicated clinician to hold and protect the placement of the ETT.

Transport Specific Ventilators

Equipment Selection

Modes in the transport ventilators all have proprietary names but serve similar functions. As highlighted in Chap. 8, these variations mandate that clinicians familiarize themselves with the transport ventilator used by their service prior to transporting patients. There are relatively few transport ventilators available capable of

Table 16.3 Weight limits for neonatal and pediatric ventilator equipment

Ventilator	Neonate/infant	Pediatric
Hamilton T1	0.2–30 kg	Up to 48 kg
Zoll Z	5–10 kg	10–40 kg
CareFusion ReVel	5 kg minimum	>5 kg

providing invasive ventilator support throughout all age/size ranges from within the pediatric patient population, and familiarity with the limits of a particular ventilator is crucial to safely support pediatric patients.

Additionally, smaller pediatric patients may *not* be appropriate for adult or universal-size equipment such as circuits, flow sensors, and $EtCO_2$ monitoring due to dead-space creation, inability to sense accurately at low volumes, and weight. Familiarity with organizational equipment and limitations is crucial to minimize negative effects to pediatric patients. Table 16.3 includes patient limitations of the three most common critical care transport ventilators available in the United States. Pediatric specific transport ventilators are also available but are beyond the scope of this review.

Table 16.3 provides weight limits for various ventilators.

References

1. Losek JD, Olson LR, Dobson JV, Glaeser PW. Tracheal intubation practice and maintaining skill competency: survey of pediatric emergency department medical directors. Pediatr Emerg Care. 2008;24(5):294–9. https://doi.org/10.1097/PEC.0B013E31816ECBD4.
2. Kollisch-Singule M, Ramcharran H, Satalin J, et al. Mechanical ventilation in pediatric and neonatal patients. Front Physiol. 2022;12:12. https://doi.org/10.3389/FPHYS.2021.805620.
3. Saikia D, Mahanta B. Cardiovascular and respiratory physiology in children. Indian J Anaesth. 2019;63(9):690. https://doi.org/10.4103/ija.IJA_490_19.
4. Lyng J, Harris M, Mandt M, et al. Prehospital pediatric respiratory distress and airway management training and education: an NAEMSP position statement and resource document. Prehosp Emerg Care. 2022;26(S1):102. https://doi.org/10.1080/10903127.2021.1992551.
5. Cheifetz IM. Invasive and noninvasive pediatric mechanical ventilation. Respir Care. 2003;48(4):442.
6. Jouvet P, Thomas NJ, Willson DF, et al. Pediatric acute respiratory distress syndrome: consensus recommendations from the pediatric acute lung injury consensus conference. Pediatr Crit Care Med. 2015;16(5):428–39. https://doi.org/10.1097/PCC.0000000000000350.
7. Kneyber MCJ, de Luca D, Calderini E, et al. Recommendations for mechanical ventilation of critically ill children from the Paediatric mechanical ventilation consensus conference (PEMVECC). Intensive Care Med. 2017;43:1764. https://doi.org/10.1007/s00134-017-4920-z.
8. The Acute Respiratory Distress Syndrome Network. Ventilation with lower tidal volumes as compared with traditional tidal volumes for acute lung injury and the acute respiratory distress syndrome. N Engl J Med. 2000;342(18):1301–8. https://doi.org/10.1056/NEJM200005043421801.
9. Smallwood CD, Davis MD. Year in review 2018: pediatric mechanical ventilation. Respir Care. 2019;64(7):855–63. https://doi.org/10.4187/RESPCARE.07029.
10. Muniraman HK, Song AY, Ramanathan R, et al. Evaluation of oxygen saturation index compared with oxygenation index in neonates with hypoxemic respiratory failure. JAMA Netw Open. 2019;2(3):e191179. https://doi.org/10.1001/JAMANETWORKOPEN.2019.1179.

17 Mechanical Ventilation for Neonatal Transport

Jamie Eastman and Michael Prendergast

Neonatal Specific Physiology and Pathophysiology

Transition from Fetal Circulation to Neonatal Circulation

At birth, the cardiopulmonary circulation transitions from the fetus' dependence on the placenta to independent pulmonary gas exchange in the healthy newborn. Lung inflation causes pulmonary vasodilation, decreasing pulmonary vascular resistance and facilitating blood flow through the lungs to establish the lungs as the site of gas exchange. The consequent increase in pulmonary venous return raises the left atrial pressure, which functionally closes the patent foramen ovale (PFO), reducing right-to-left shunting at the atrial level. The higher oxygen levels and prostaglandin clearance facilitate the ductus arteriosus's closure, reducing right-to-left shunting at the ductal level. Removal of the low-resistance placenta from circulation increases systemic vascular resistance. The combination of decreased pulmonary vascular resistance, increased systemic vascular resistance, and closure of pathways for right-to-left shunting contributes to establishing pulmonary blood flow and gas exchange. Factors interfering with these critical physiological changes, e.g., meconium pneumonitis, may result in a delayed drop in pulmonary vascular resistance and result in persistent fetal circulation.

Patent Ductus Arteriosus (PDA)

Closure of the ductus arteriosus typically occurs within 12–72 h of birth in term newborns. In premature infants, the mechanism for ductus arteriosus closure is

J. Eastman · M. Prendergast (✉)
Boston MedFlight, Bedford, MA, USA

St. Elizabeth's Medical Center, Brighton, MA, USA
e-mail: jamie.eastman@bostonmedflight.org; mprendergast2@mgh.harvard.edu

© The Author(s), under exclusive license to Springer Nature Switzerland AG 2024

S. R. Wilcox et al. (eds.), *Mechanical Ventilation in Critical Care Transport*,
https://doi.org/10.1007/978-3-031-66782-4_17

poorly developed, causing it to remain patent at times. As the pulmonary vascular resistance drops postnatally, blood may be shunted from the aorta, across the PDA, to the pulmonary arteries. This increased pulmonary blood flow predisposes to pulmonary edema, which may lead to worsening pulmonary mechanics, impaired gas exchange, and increased ventilatory and cardiac workload.

Airway

The neonatal airway has several anatomical distinctions (e.g., heavy head relative to poor neck mobility, narrow trachea, underdeveloped cartilaginous support of the trachea) that make it more susceptible to obstruction than children or adults. In noninvasive MV support, attention should be paid to head/neck positioning, using a shoulder/neck roll where necessary. Small degrees of endotracheal tube (ETT) movement for intubated infants can result in extubation or main stem intubation. Therefore, the ETT position should be verified clinically and by X-ray and secured for transport. Where an ETT cannot be placed, a laryngeal mask airway may be considered in late preterm infants and term infants.

Surfactant and Lung Physiology

Surfactant is a lipid-protein compound that is secreted into the alveoli. It lowers the surface tension of alveoli, reducing their tendency to collapse, which facilitates the establishment of functional residual capacity (FRC) and reduces the pressure needed to inflate alveoli. Impaired surfactant production (e.g., in prematurity) and activity (e.g., in meconium aspiration syndrome) results in poorly compliant lungs prone to atelectasis. Administration of antenatal steroids can accelerate surfactant production.

Chest wall compliance is significantly higher in newborns, especially premature newborns, than in children or adults. The compliant chest wall retracts with the negative pressure generated by diaphragmatic contractions during inspiration which exacerbates the tendency for atelectasis. In the term newborn, the airway diameter is much less than in adults; thus, the airway resistance is significantly greater.

The combination of low lung compliance, high chest wall compliance, and high airway resistance contributes to a high work of breathing in newborns, particularly premature newborns in whom these factors are more pronounced.

Oxygen Therapy and Toxicity

Supplemental oxygen is frequently used to achieve adequate tissue oxygenation in newborns; however, oxygen may cause oxidative stress and generate reactive oxygen species. Preterm infants have an immature antioxidant defense system and so are especially vulnerable to such injury, which contributes significantly to major morbidities such as retinopathy of prematurity (ROP), bronchopulmonary dysplasia (BPD), and periventricular leukomalacia (PVL). Striking a balance between the risks and benefits of O_2 therapy in preterm infants is challenging. Using a lower (85–89%) versus a higher (91–95%) SpO_2 target range in extremely premature infants is associated with higher mortality and necrotizing enterocolitis (NEC) but a lower risk of ROP and BPD [1]. The optimal SpO_2 target range for more mature infants is also uncertain. Therefore, this should be a discussion point for transport teams for each mechanically ventilated neonate.

Respiratory support needs may differ between neonatal patients and within the same patient over time. This is particularly true in preterm infants when cardiorespiratory physiology (e.g., pulmonary dynamics, circulation) changes rapidly. Individualized assessment, patient-specific ventilator modes and settings selection, and frequent reassessment are necessary.

Ventilator Induced Lung Injury (VILI)

Though mechanical ventilation is often a critical support, it also risks injury to the developing lungs (e.g., volutrauma, barotrauma, atelectrauma, hyperoxia). It impacts hemodynamics with the potential for adverse effects on the brain and other organs. While mechanical ventilation can induce injury in any patient, the MV protective strategies are particularly important in preterm newborns to avoid key morbidities such as BPD, ROP, IVH, and PVL.

Altitude Physiology

Neonates have several unique anatomical and physiological characteristics potentially sensitive to altitude. The alveolar-arterial oxygen difference in neonates (approximately 25 mmHg) is typically much larger than in adults (approximately 10 mmHg) [2]. Therefore, a modest drop in partial pressure of alveolar oxygen during ascent may result in hypoxia in neonates, especially preterm neonates, with the result that the baby must work harder to achieve satisfactory gas exchange. This highlights the need for close monitoring and anticipating the need for increasing support as altitude increases.

As altitude increases and barometric pressure consequently decreases, gas expansion may occur in the neonate, most notably in the gastrointestinal tract, which may exacerbate respiratory distress by impinging on the diaphragm. This can be mitigated by using a naso- / oro-gastric tube to decompress the gastrointestinal tract in infants on mechanical ventilation. Similarly, the potential for gas expansion should be considered when transporting an infant with a pneumothorax, perhaps prompting earlier intervention than would usually be required.

Noninvasive Mechanical Ventilation

Where appropriate, noninvasive ventilator support is preferentially used to minimize VILI. Nasal prongs are the preferred interface. A RAM nasal cannula (NeoTech, Valencia, California) has larger bore tubing than a typical nasal cannula, thereby reducing resistance and the work of breathing. RAM cannulas have no expiratory limb, so expiration occurs through the leaks at the nose and mouth instead, delivering a pressure less than the set value.

A pacifier or chin strap may help if an open mouth creates a large leak. Infants on noninvasive MV, particularly term or late preterm infants who can generate strong exhalation force against CPAP, are at risk for thoracic air leaks leading to pneumothoraces.

An orogastric tube should be placed alongside noninvasive ventilation to minimize GI distension [2, 3].

Continuous Positive Airway Pressure (CPAP)

CPAP pressure is typically started at 5–7 cm H_2O and then adjusted according to breathing work or signs of over−/underinflation.

Noninvasive Intermittent Positive Pressure Ventilation

Newborns who require acute transport for respiratory disease that is refractory to CPAP are typically intubated for invasive MV. However, NIPPV may be used after birth to minimize invasive VILI or later in the neonatal course after extubation from invasive MV. NIPPV is contraindicated in infants with upper airway abnormalities such as cleft palate.

Invasive Mechanical Ventilation

Conventional Mechanical Ventilation

In newborns, volume-targeted ventilation (VTV) is preferred for its consistent volume delivery despite changing lung compliance. Typical initial settings include tidal volume (Vt) of 4–6 mL/kg to avoid volutrauma/barotrauma, PEEP of 5–6 cm H_2O to avoid atelectrauma, and an inspiratory time (Ti) of 0.35–0.4 s, as shown in Fig. 17.1.

Accurate Vt measurement is critical for VTV; however, this may be challenging due to air leaks around uncuffed ETTs in neonates, in which case pressure-limited ventilation is used.

Effective Vt is affected by equipment dead space, e.g., ETT, and physiologic dead space in respiratory disease, e.g., BPD. In smaller preterm babies with a

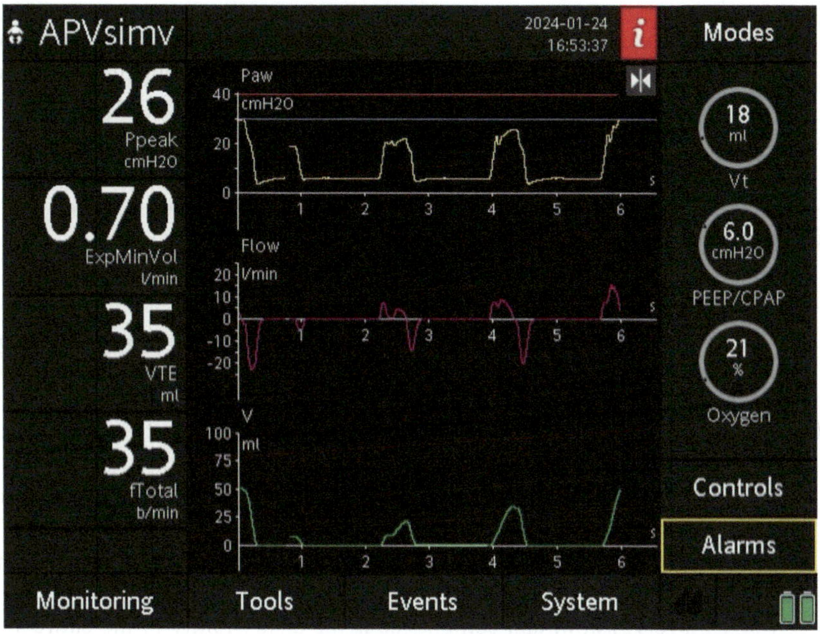

Fig. 17.1 A ventilator screen of a neonate. The TV is set at 18 mL, and the patient has just exhaled 35 mL. The rate is 35, the PEEP is 6 cmH_2O, and the FiO_2 is 21%

weight-based Vt target, the proportion of the total Vt that is delivered to the lungs decreases due to the proportionally larger fixed dead space; therefore, a larger set Vt may be considered.

Adjusting PIP based on lung compliance is important in pressure-limited ventilation. This is particularly important in preterm infants after surfactant treatment.

When using SIMV, PS should be added to provide enough Vt to overcome dead space and prevent increased work of breathing.

High-Frequency Oscillatory Ventilation

High-frequency oscillatory ventilation (HFOV) uses pressure oscillations to deliver rapid-rate, low Vt around a constant distending mean airway pressure. It may be used in the NICU as a primary mode or as a rescue mode in the setting of respiratory failure that is refractory to conventional mechanical ventilation (CMV).

Lung inflation supports lung recruitment for oxygenation. Excessive lung inflation may cause decreasing venous return and compromise cardiac output, while underinflation may cause atelectasis and hypoxemia. The amplitude of oscillations controls CO_2 clearance.

Though high-frequency oscillatory ventilators for infant transport are commercially available, this mode of MV is not consistently carried or used by neonatal transport teams. Therefore, babies typically transition from HFOV to CMV for transport using a MAP 2 cm H_2O less than that used for HFOV. Transition to CMV as far in advance of transport as possible, and check a blood gas and chest X-ray after approximately 30 min. If a baby on HFOV cannot be stabilized after transition to CMV, undertaking transport may be ill-advised.

Adjunct Therapies

Inhaled Nitric Oxide

Inhaled nitric oxide (iNO) is a potent and selective pulmonary vasodilator which improves blood flow to the well-ventilated areas of the lung, improving ventilation-perfusion mismatch in term and near-term newborns with PPHN. It is administered via the ventilator circuit at a rate of 20 parts per million. If oxygenation improves in response to iNO, inspired FiO_2 is weaned. Weaning iNO is a gradual process that should be avoided on transport, even in nonresponders, to minimize the risk of rebound pulmonary hypertension.

Exogenous Surfactant

Exogenous surfactant may be administered endotracheally to preterm and occasionally term infants with respiratory distress within the first day of life. In the context of neonatal transport, newborns are typically intubated for surfactant administration and placed on MV for transport. However, in clinically appropriate cases, infants may be immediately extubated and placed on CPAP after surfactant to provide the therapeutic benefit of surfactant while avoiding the potential side effects of MV. Lung compliance changes should be anticipated during the first 30 min following administration and ventilator settings adjusted accordingly. Potential adverse effects include pulmonary air leaks and pulmonary hemorrhage.

Common Neonatal Clinical Conditions Requiring Mechanical Ventilation

Respiratory Distress Syndrome

This is primarily a complication of prematurity due to surfactant deficiency, which causes widespread atelectasis leading to increased work of breathing, ventilation-perfusion mismatch, and poor gas exchange [4]. The diagnosis is based on clinical respiratory distress and X-ray findings of diffuse atelectasis (Fig. 17.2).

Affected infants require distending pressure support to inflate alveoli [4]. If there is reasonable spontaneous respiratory effort and only mild hypercapnia, the use of

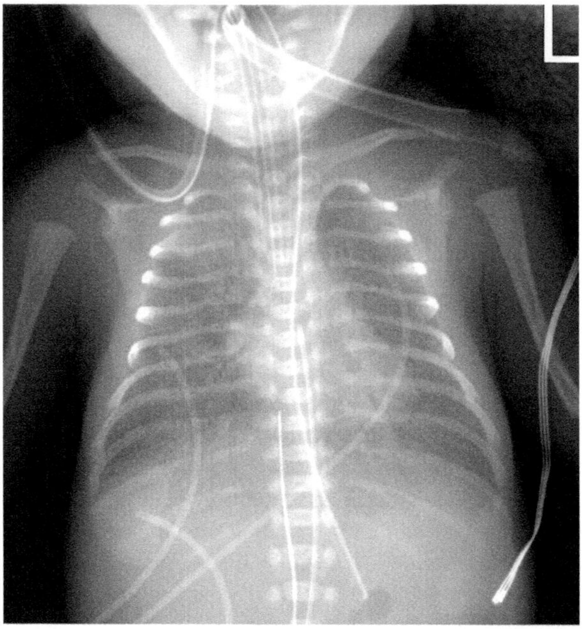

Fig. 17.2 Chest X-Ray of preterm newborn demonstrating the "ground-glass" appearance of the lung fields characteristic of surfactant deficiency

CPAP is preferable for this purpose. However, if noninvasive MV is insufficient and respiratory distress, inadequate gas exchange (e.g., $FiO_2 > 0.3$ on CPAP 6 cm H_2O; $PaCO_2 > 65$ mmHg), and reduced respiratory drive persist, the infant should be intubated for surfactant administration and invasive MV using lung protective strategies. Settings should be adjusted based on clinical assessment, FiO_2 requirement, chest radiographs, and blood gas analysis as needed. Modest permissive hypercapnia (pCO_2 40–65 mmHg) may be tolerated.

Meconium Aspiration Syndrome (MAS)

Aspiration of meconium in amniotic fluid may cause airway obstruction (with air trapping and air leak syndrome), chemical pneumonitis, lung inflammation, and surfactant inactivation. Clinical presentation is characterized by early and progressive respiratory distress and hypoxemia. X-ray findings include bilateral patchy infiltrates and increased lung volumes due to gas trapping. Affected infants are at risk of persistent pulmonary hypertension and air leaks.

Infants with moderate-severe disease should be intubated, given surfactant, and placed on a volume-targeted CMV mode to achieve adequate gas exchange for transport while minimizing VILI. Use supplemental FiO_2 as required and mild permissive hypercapnia may be allowed, but pH should be kept in the normal range to avoid exacerbating pulmonary hypertension.

Persistent Pulmonary Hypertension of the Newborn (PPHN)

Disruption in the normal transition from fetal to neonatal circulation may result in sustained elevation of pulmonary vascular resistance and right-to-left shunting of blood via the PDA and/or patent foramen ovale (PFO) causing hypoxemia. It can be idiopathic or associated with respiratory diseases, e.g., MAS. The clinical diagnosis is challenging as it may occur in the absence of respiratory distress, a pre- and post-ductal oxygenation difference, or radiographic evidence of an underlying pulmonary disorder. An echocardiogram demonstrating elevated pulmonary pressures with right-to-left shunting is ultimately required for diagnosis.

The first step is to treat any underlying cause of the delayed physiologic transition. Invasive MV is required for clinically significant PPHN. Lung recruitment is achieved by gentle ventilation strategies using PEEP, relatively low PIP or Vt, and a degree of permissive hypercapnia to ensure adequate lung expansion while limiting barotrauma and volutrauma. Once lung recruitment has been optimized, further management should be based on oxygenation status. Surfactant may be beneficial. The Oxygenation Index [(mean airway pressure × FiO_2)/(PaO_2 in mmHg × 100)] is a commonly used score to guide further intervention such as the use of iNO. Sedation should be used routinely, and neuromuscular blockade should be considered. Systemic vascular resistance should be supported with IV volume or vasopressors.

Pneumothorax

Pneumothoraces can occur spontaneously; however, most occur in association with uneven ventilation, alveolar overdistention, and air trapping. Risk factors include both underlying pulmonary diseases, e.g., pulmonary hypoplasia, and the MV settings used to provide respiratory support (long inspiratory time, high CPAP or PIP, and large Vt). The typical clinical presentation is with respiratory distress, increased FiO_2, asymmetric breath sounds, and hemodynamic compromise. Increased transmission of light on transillumination of the affected hemithorax may help detect a pneumothorax; however, transport teams should obtain a chest X-ray prior to transport of infants with respiratory distress and any concern for air leak/pneumothorax, particularly if planned to go to elevated altitude.

In infants who are on MV, minimizing the mean airway pressure will help offset the air leak. Treatment of a pneumothorax before transport will depend on the size of the air leak. A moderate pneumothorax may be treated with needle thoracentesis; however, chest tube placement may be required for a large pneumothorax prior to transport.

Pulmonary Hemorrhage

Left to right shunting through a PDA in premature infants or congestive heart failure may increase capillary pressure in the pulmonary interstitial space causing bloody edema to leak into alveoli. This presents as fresh blood or blood-tinged secretions in the ETT, increased work of breathing, and increased ventilatory requirements.

If not already intubated, place an ETT. Increase CMV settings to provide a higher MAP to stabilize lung volume and suppress further hemorrhage. Consider endotracheal administration of epinephrine to stop the bleeding, and provide hemodynamic support using blood products, if available, and pressor medication.

Congenital Diaphragmatic Hernia (CDH)

It is a developmental defect of the diaphragm that allows abdominal viscera to herniate into the chest. It can be associated with other congenital anomalies, e.g., cardiac disease, which should be considered in medical management during transport. Affected infants are at risk for air leaks and pulmonary hypertension, especially in the case of marked pulmonary hypoplasia.

Infants with CDH should be promptly intubated after birth without mask ventilation, along with placement of a large orogastric tube to suction, to prevent gaseous distention of herniated bowel. A gentle ventilation strategy using pressure-limited ventilation settings to minimize barotrauma (PIP <25 cm H2O) should be used. Gas exchange targets should include permissive hypercapnia (pCO_2 50–60 mmHg, once pH remains >7.25) and a preductal SpO_2 target range of 85–95%. Monitor for and support PPHN where present.

Bronchopulmonary Dysplasia (BPD)

BPD is a major morbidity of prematurity caused by both injury to and maldevelopment of the lungs leading to fewer, larger alveoli with less surface area for gas exchange. Clinical findings include hypoxia and respiratory distress requiring supplemental oxygen and MV support. Affected infants are at risk for airway hyperresponsiveness and pulmonary hypertension.

The MV management of BPD is aimed at maintaining adequate gas exchange while limiting the progression of lung damage. One major challenge is that the MV and supplemental oxygen required to maintain gas exchange are also key factors implicated in the progression of lung damage. Noninvasive support is preferable where possible, although higher CPAP of 6–10 cm H_2O may be required. Where invasive MV is required, high PEEP levels can help reduce expiratory airway resistance and gas trapping and improve alveolar ventilation, while the lowest peak airway pressures to deliver adequate Vt should be used along with longer inspiratory times of 0.4–0.6 s to improve distribution of inspired gas. In severe BPD, the ratio of dead space to Vt increases which reduces effective ventilation so a higher Vt (6–10 mL/kg) may be required. Target oxygen saturation ranges are center specific, and higher degrees of permissive hypercapnia are commonly accepted once pH is in the normal range.

Congenital Heart Disease

There are many different forms of congenital cardiac disease, broadly categorized as either cyanotic or acyanotic conditions. Differentiating hypoxia due to cyanotic cardiac disease or pulmonary disease is clinically challenging. Physical examination, chest X-ray, and hyperoxia test are important, but echocardiography is required to establish a diagnosis and management plan.

Where cyanosis persists despite optimal MV strategies and maximal supplemental oxygen, cyanotic heart disease should be suspected. Consider starting prostaglandin E1 (PGE1) infusion immediately, regardless of availability of a definitive diagnosis. The approach to MV and oxygen management depends on the cardiac lesion of concern and should be determined with input from an expert in neonatal medicine.

Airway Protection and/or Reduced Respiratory Drive

MV may be required for transport in the context of endotracheal intubation for neonatal airway protection (e.g., tracheomalacia, congenital airway malformations such as Pierre-Robin sequence) or reduced respiratory drive (e.g., apnea of prematurity, seizures, respiratory depression medication side effects).

CPAP may be sufficient in infants with upper airway abnormalities predisposing to narrowing or collapse; however, invasive mechanical ventilation may be required in more severe cases of airway abnormality and those with insufficient respiratory drive. Pressure support alone may be used in patients with adequate respiratory drive; otherwise, a set rate is required. Set volume and pressure support requirements should be minimal given the lack of pulmonary disease.

References

1. Askie LM, Darlow BA, Finer N, Schmidt B, Stenson B, Tarnow-Mordi W, Davis PG, Carlo WA, Brocklehurst P, Davies LC, Das A, Rich W, Gantz MG, Roberts RS, Whyte RK, Costantini L, Poets C, Asztalos E, Battin M, Halliday HL, Marlow N, Tin W, King A, Juszczak E, Morley CJ, Doyle LW, Gebski V, Hunter KE, Simes RJ, Neonatal Oxygenation Prospective Meta-analysis (NeOProM) Collaboration. Association between oxygen saturation targeting and death or disability in extremely preterm infants in the neonatal oxygenation prospective meta-analysis collaboration. JAMA. 2018;319(21):2190–201.
2. Meyer K, Fernandes CJ, Schwartz HP. AAP section on transport medicine. Neonatal content. Field guide for air and ground transport of neonatal and pediatric patients. 2018.
3. Brennan G, Colontuono J, Carlos C. Neonatal respiratory support on transport. NeoReviews. 2019;20(4):e202–12.
4. Donn SM, Mammel MC, van Kaam AHLC. Manual of neonatal respiratory care. Cham: Springer; 2022.

Responding to Ventilator Alarms 18

Vahé Ender

Introduction

Despite the inherent goal of acting as safeguards against patient injury, ventilator alarms pose a significant challenge to patient safety due to their mixed levels of importance—while some may represent an easily correctible problem, others may be the sign of an immediate life threat that could be fatal if left unaddressed promptly.

In the often chaotic critical care transport environment, rife with audible chimes and alerts, efforts have been made to decrease alarm fatigue by providing tiered alarms on medical devices based on their relative severity. This text aims to accomplish the same by providing a structured approach to ventilator troubleshooting.

The most important concept when caring for a ventilated patient is that no alarm is generated by the ventilator without reason, and *all* alarms are an indication of a problem requiring clinician evaluation. The only difference between a lower severity alarm and one indicating a life threat is *how quickly one must act.*

In the event of any alarm, initial assessments must be made to determine the seriousness of the alarm. This can be done by simple assessments of both the patient and the ventilator. These exams focus on the determination of whether the alarm is an indication of it no longer providing life support or if the alarm is associated with patient decompensation (Tables 18.1 and 18.2).

In the event of a life-threatening emergency, a rapid response focused on identifying possible causes of patient deterioration must be undertaken. Two commonly used mnemonics can be helpful to structure this approach, with the "DOPES" mnemonic providing a means to recall causes of patient deterioration, while the "DOTTS" mnemonic provides a framework to respond to them. These are outlined in Tables 18.3 and 18.4.

V. Ender (✉)
Boston MedFlight, Bedford, MA, USA
e-mail: vahe.ender@bostonmedflight.org

© The Author(s), under exclusive license to Springer Nature Switzerland AG 2024

S. R. Wilcox et al. (eds.), *Mechanical Ventilation in Critical Care Transport*,
https://doi.org/10.1007/978-3-031-66782-4_18

Table 18.1 Signs of a life-threatening alarm on clinical exam

Inadequate chest rise and fall with each breath
Diminished lung sounds, either unilateral or bilateral
Accompanied by newly unstable vital signs
Oxygen desaturation
Absent or diminished $ETCO_2$ waveform

Table 18.2 Acutely life-threatening alarm on the ventilator

Circuit disconnect
Low oxygen alarm
Low-pressure alarm—Especially with low exhaled tidal volume
High-pressure alarm—Especially with low exhaled tidal volume

Table 18.3 DOPES mnemonic—consider differential diagnosis

Displacement	Right mainstem, extubation, herniation above the cords
Obstruction	Kinking, blood, mucous plugging
Pneumothorax	Collapse of one or both lungs
Equipment	Disconnection or malfunction
Stacking	Breath-stacking and air trapping

Table 18.4 DOTTS mnemonic—actions to assess the decompensating patient

Disconnect the patient from ventilator	Allow exhalation; remove ventilator malfunction from situation
O_2—Bag patient with 100% FiO_2 and PEEP valve at 5 cm H_2O	Assess SpO_2
Tube position	Perform exam, look for chest rise/fall bilaterally, listen for bilateral breath sounds, and assess $ETCO_2$. Pass a suction catheter to assess for and potentially clear a blockage
Tweak settings	Lower RR if needed for air trapping, increase PEEP if indicated, etc.
Scan	Ultrasound the chest (if within scope of practice) to rule out pneumothorax

Alarm Types

Ventilators generate alarms in three broad categories reviewed below:

The Device Encounters Unexpectedly Low Pressures While Providing Ventilation

Low-Pressure Alarm

In the event of an unusually *low* pressure encountered during or between breaths, the ventilator will alarm as this situation may either be a cause for derecruitment or, worse yet, be the sign of a leak between the ventilator and the patient's airway.

Low-pressure alarms can be caused by the patient's "air hunger" or inspiratory effort, which causes a negative pressure to be encountered by the vent. While providing sedation is an easy corrective action for the above scenario, a low-pressure alarm may also be due to more serious problems, including an endotracheal tube cuff leak resulting in a significant leak or malposition of the endotracheal tube into a supraglottic position (self-extubate). An endotracheal tube resting above the vocal cords at the glottic inlet has a positional loss of seal and indicates extubation. The situation that has led to the low-pressure alarm results in a loss of effective ventilation, possibly showing as low exhaled volumes or abnormalities in waveform capnography. Finally, a leak may be present at one of the connecting points along the ventilator circuit.

In circumstances where the ventilator detects a large loss of pressure which is sustained, device logic may specifically trigger a *Circuit Disconnect* alarm to alert clinicians to a possible emergent disconnection of the ventilator circuit from the patient. This feature is dependent on the ventilator model.

Low PEEP

Positive end-expiratory pressure (PEEP) is the constant pressure provided to patient lungs to prevent atelectotrauma and to optimize oxygenation. The ventilator provides this continuous pressure as the baseline from which ventilation is provided.

In circumstances where a patient has air hunger due to metabolic status or sedation levels, a large inspiratory effort can result in a loss of sustained PEEP. If this event is significant enough, the ventilator may alert with a "Low PEEP" alarm. This is shown in Fig. 18.1.

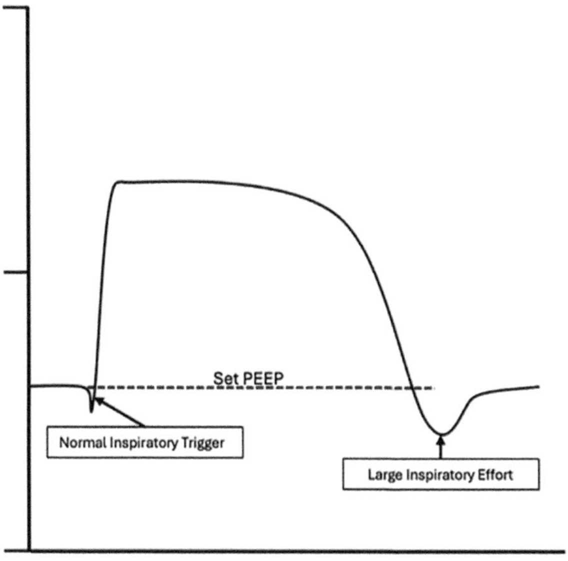

Fig. 18.1 Ventilator waveform showing a large negative deflection

The Device Encounters Abnormally High Pressures During Breath Delivery

High Pressure Limit

When delivering a breath, the airways provide a certain pressure which the ventilator must overcome. This backpressure is caused by the decreasing size of the conducting airways (trachea, bronchi, bronchioles) and having to deliver a set tidal volume to the alveoli. An important concept to remember is that the "High Pressure" alarm is a *limit*. This is shown in Fig. 18.2. If the high-pressure threshold is reached during breath delivery, the breath will be terminated, and the desired tidal volumes may not be reached. This could result in a decreased minute ventilation if allowed to continue. To determine if ventilation is being impaired, monitor the exhaled volumes on the ventilator (Fig. 18.2).

The peak inspiratory pressure (PIP) is the maximal pressure generated during delivery of the breath. This is the result of two phenomena: resistance and compliance (see Chaps. 3, 7, and 10). *Resistance* is caused by a backpressure generated by the circuit, ETT, and the conducting airways during breath delivery and does not reflect the intra-alveolar pressure. An elevated resistance can be due to a circuit obstruction, saturation of a heat-moisture exchanger, mucus plug, or bronchospasm.

High peak pressures due to poor *compliance* reflect lung disease of the parenchyma and alveoli or by way of external compression of the lungs by high intrapleural pressures. This pressure can be generated within the lung by worsening disease

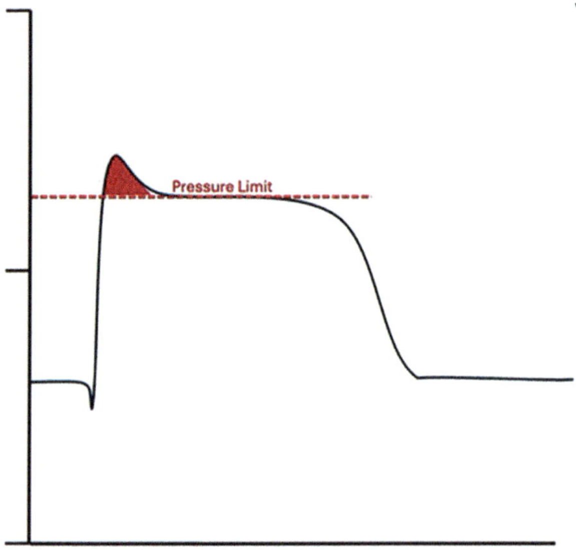

Fig. 18.2 A waveform indicating a high pressure limit

such as ARDS, pulmonary edema. High airway pressures can also be the result of accumulation of pressure within the lung due to air trapping. This phenomenon, referred to as breath-stacking, causes for a gradual decrease in functional residual capacity due to retained ventilated volumes trapped by bronchospasm.

Differentiating a resistance problem versus a compliance problem is simple with many modern ventilators. They may provide continuous, dynamic resistance and compliance values. Some ventilators may require a measurement of the plateau pressure (Pplat) to measure the intra-alveolar pressures after breath delivery—a high Pplat indicates high pressure within the lung parenchyma and a problem of lung compliance. If the difference between the peak inspiratory pressure and the plateau pressure is greater than 5 cmH_2O, this indicates a problem of resistance (see Chap. 3), as is shown in Fig. 18.3. Figure 18.4 demonstrates low compliance.

Following a high-pressure limit, an evaluation must be made from patient-to-ventilator to identify the cause, following the DOPES and DOTTS mnemonics. This is illustrated in Fig. 18.5.

Patient comfort must be assessed to determine whether the high pressures are due to coughing or asynchrony. The endotracheal tube should be evaluated to whether the patient is biting down on the airway or if there is a kink. A soft suction catheter can be passed to assess for secretions or a mucus obstruction causing resistance to flow. Auscultation of lung sounds may reveal a cause for high airway resistance such as bronchospasm, aspiration, pneumothorax, or pulmonary edema.

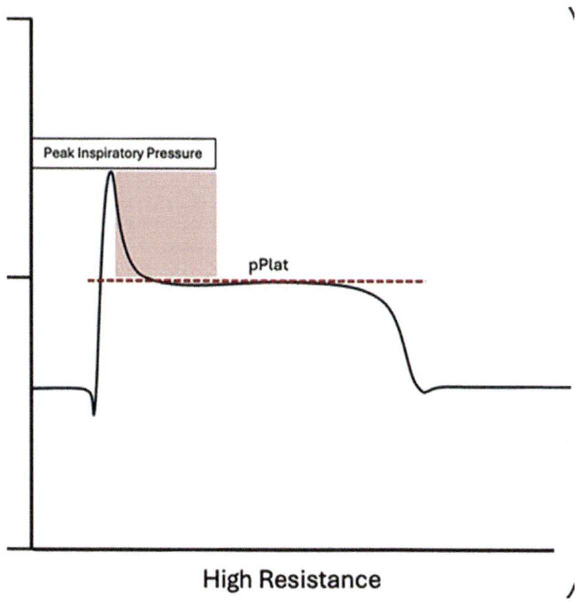

Fig. 18.3 The large difference between the peak inspiratory pressure (PIP) and the plateau pressure indicates a problem of resistance

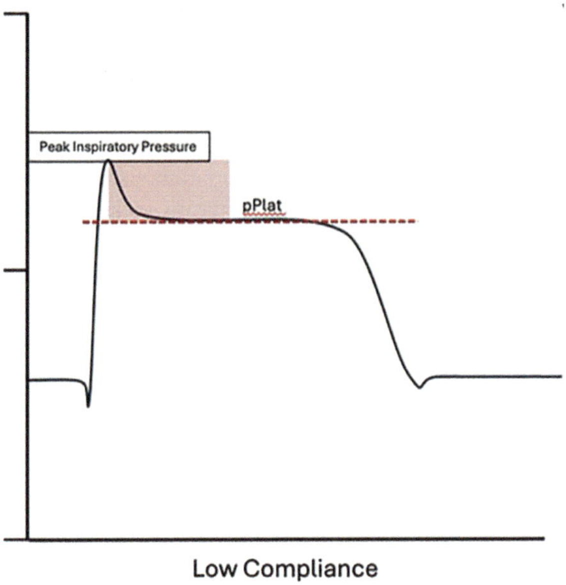

Fig. 18.4 The high pressures with a low difference between the PIP and the plateau shows an issue with complaince

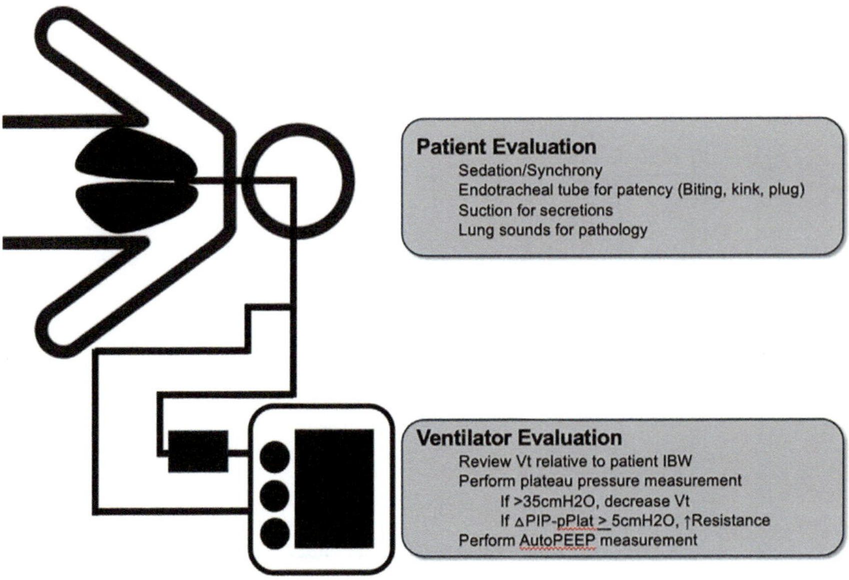

Fig. 18.5 Clinicians should work from the patient towards the ventilator, systematically checking each component for a potentially life-threatening cause of a ventilator alarm

From there, the ventilator must be surveyed to further guide the management of high pressures. In cases where mechanical ventilation has been initiated prior to clinician arrival, tidal volumes being delivered should be compared relative to the patient ideal body weight (IBW) to determine whether the volumes are potentially the cause of high pressures.

Another potential cause for a "high-pressure" alarm is breath-stacking at times due to autoPEEP. To identify the possibility of breath-stacking, measuring the residual pressure after exhalation and comparing it to the set PEEP level will reveal any remaining volume being retained. In some ventilators, this may trigger a "High PEEP" alarm, as the device is sensing an end-expiratory pressure above what is set by the clinician.

The Device Is Seeing Ventilation Trends Falling Outside of Settings for Surveillance

Ventilators can be configured to provide alarms to alert clinicians to a developing trend. These are generally lower-tier alarms but can provide early warning of changes in patient condition. Though considered a nuisance by some, these settings allow for safer ventilation and should be set with patient protection in mind.

Settings that will generally alert staff to an early development of increase in respiratory effort or air hunger are "High f," "High Tidal Volume," and the sum of the two, "High Minute Ventilation."

These can provide early warning of a patient being subject to lightening sedation before the patient may become asynchronous and trigger a high-pressure alarm. As with other issues in medicine, early intervention results in the avoidance of more serious events with greater consequence.

Further Reading

Santanilla JI, Daniel B, Yeow ME. Mechanical ventilation. Emerg Med Clin North Am. 2008;26(3):849–62.

Thomas VK, Abraham SV. Adding an "R" in the "DOPE" mnemonic for ventilator troubleshooting. Indian J Crit Care Med. 2018;22(5):388.

Case Studies in Mechanical Ventilation

19

James Rawson and Susan R. Wilcox

Case 1

A 40-year-old man with a history of alcohol use disorder and decompensated cirrhosis, with a recent hospitalization for spontaneous bacterial peritonitis, returns to the ED. He arrived with a several days' history of fatigue and increasing abdominal girth. Patient notes that he has had recent alcohol consumption but otherwise poor oral intake. He denies pain but states that he has had melanotic stools and had one episode of bloody emesis this morning. The patient is tachycardic, with a heart rate of 120, is hypotensive with a blood pressure of 98/53 mmHg, and has SpO_2 ~ 88% on room air, improving only to 92% with a nonrebreather. His cardiac exam is regular, and breath sounds are diminished throughout. His abdomen is large, distended, but not tender to palpation. He has WBC of 22, Hgb of 6.6, and lactate of 3.7. His chest X-ray is shown in Fig. 19.1.

1. Why might this patient be hypoxemic?
2. What are your airway concerns with this patient?
   The patient becomes more hypoxemic and tachypneic and is intubated for hypoxemia and airway protection.
3. What would you expect to encounter once this patient is placed on the ventilator?
   His ventilator screen is shown in Fig. 19.2.
   The team performs an inspiratory hold to assess for compliance and resistance, shown in Fig. 19.3.
4. What is your assessment of the patient's compliance? Is this more of a resistance or a compliance issue?
5. A blood gas is drawn, and the patient's P/F ratio is 112—what is the significance of this?

J. Rawson · S. R. Wilcox (✉)
Boston MedFlight, Bedford, MA, USA
e-mail: susan.r.wilcox@lahey.org

© The Author(s), under exclusive license to Springer Nature Switzerland AG 2024

S. R. Wilcox et al. (eds.), *Mechanical Ventilation in Critical Care Transport*,
https://doi.org/10.1007/978-3-031-66782-4_19

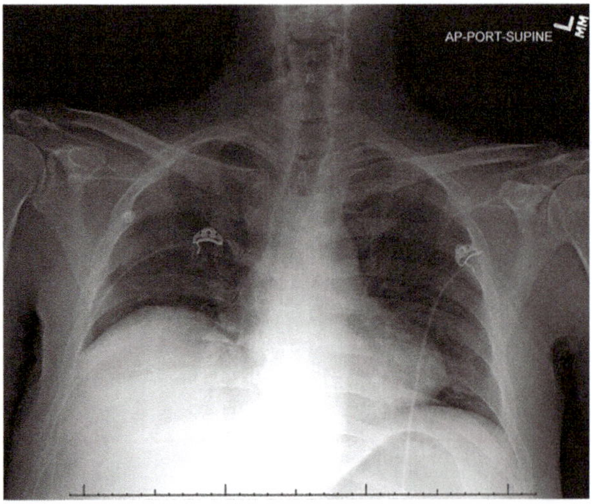

Fig. 19.1 Chest X-ray for Case 1

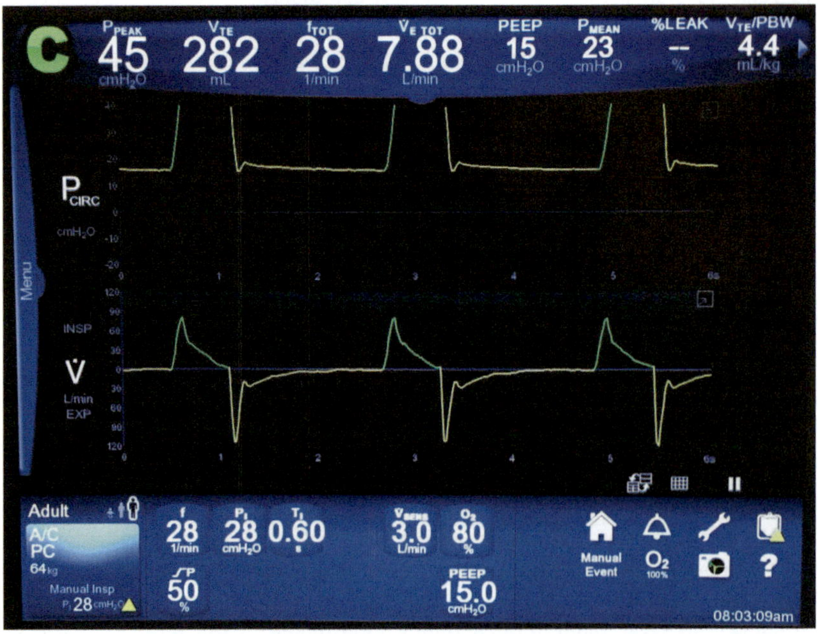

Fig. 19.2 Ventilator screen for Case 1

6. What options or adjuncts do you have for increasing the oxygenation of this patient?
7. What ventilator strategies would you use for ventilating this patient?
8. What are the current ventilator settings? How would you describe these to your partner?

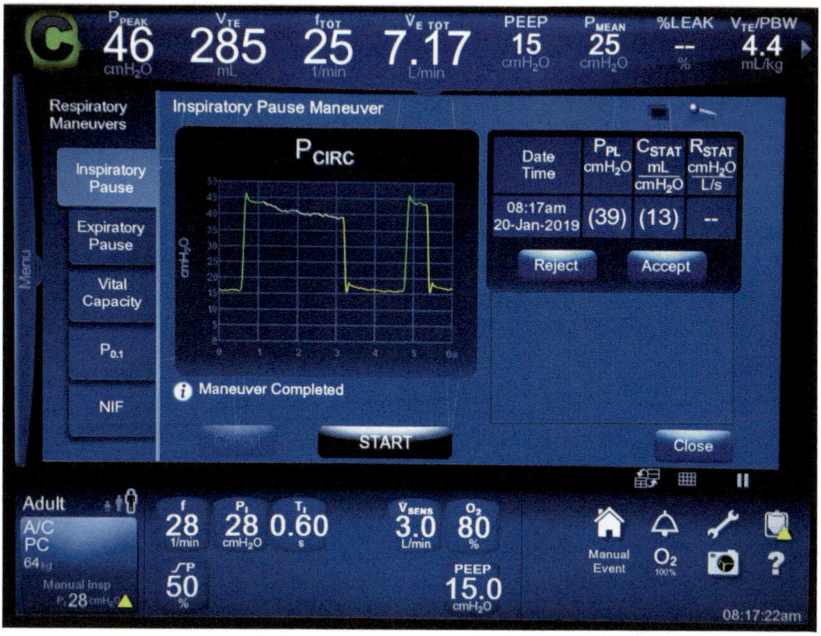

Fig. 19.3 Second ventilator screen for Case 5

Case 1 Answers

1. This patient may have many reasons to be hypoxic; however, there are two possible causes that are most likely in this clinical scenario. The first is that the patient has evidence of a swollen, distended abdomen. Increasing intra-abdominal pressure can reduce the excursion of the diaphragm leading to a decrease in alveolar ventilation. This can result in hypoxemia if the patient is not able to take a full breath. This mechanism is also supported by the patient's chest X-ray, demonstrating elevated diaphragms. Another common mechanism is aspiration. Patients with a GI bleed, especially in the setting of alcohol or other substance use, are at risk for aspiration. While the patient's chest X-ray does not demonstrate aspiration, the radiographic appearance may be delayed.
2. Immediate airway concerns for this patient include active GI bleed. Patients with a history of cirrhosis are at high risk of GI bleeds from many mechanisms, specifically esophageal varices, but also gastric ulcers, duodenal ulcers, gastritis, and Dieulafoy lesions. Any of these pathologies leading to bleeding can result in aspiration. Securing this patient's airway in the setting of respiratory failure should be a priority to avoid aspiration and worsening hypoxia. Noninvasive ventilation should not be used.
3. Increased PIP, worsening compliance, and increased resistance.
4. The PIP is 46 cmH_2O and the Pplat is 39. This patient has a very mild resistance problem (PIP—Pplat >5.) In this case, it is 7. However, the compliance issue is

far worse than the resistance issue. The compliance is 13, which is about 87 points below normal. Here, the ventilator calculates it for you, but it can be calculated as the change in volume (285 mL)/the change in pressure (Pplat—PEEP) = (39–15).

285/24 ≈ 12, or very close to the 13 from the ventilator.

5. A P/F of 112 indicates moderate to severe hypoxemia.
6. Typically, the options are to paralyze, prone the patient, or initiate inhaled pulmonary vasodilators. In this circumstance, the primary mechanisms of hypoxemia are alveolar hypoventilation and shunt from collapsed alveoli at the bases with the increased abdominal pressure. Releasing the abdominal compartment syndrome (via laparotomy) is essential to allow for full ventilation and reduction of shunting.
7. Lower volumes and higher respiratory rates. Increased PEEP.
8. The mode is AC/PC, 28/15 PEEP, rate 28 breaths per minute, 80% FiO_2. With the poor compliance, the tidal volumes are extremely low, at 270–280 mls.

Case 2

A 36-year-old woman with a long history of severe asthma presented to a local emergency department for a persistent asthma flare. Despite receiving all appropriate medical therapy, the patient continued to deteriorate with a high work of breathing. As the patient was beginning to tire out clinically, her arterial blood gas was 7.25/56/130. The emergency department staff intubated her prior to transport. The transport team arrives to take her to a tertiary care center, and they encounter this ventilator screen, as shown in Fig. 19.4.

1. What are indications to intubate a patient during an asthma exacerbation? What are the risks?
2. In what mode is this patient being ventilated?
3. What is the tidal volume? What is the respiratory rate?

   In this case, the well-intentioned team turned up the respiratory rate to address the patient's respiratory acidosis prior to the intubation. The patient then became hypotensive, with a heart rate of 110 beats per minute and a blood pressure of 88/68 mmHg. The team checked for autoPEEP, as shown on the ventilator screen on Fig. 19.5.
4. What is the autoPEEP? What is the clinical significance of this finding?
5. How should the team proceed now?
6. What is the general approach for managing a ventilator in a patient with asthma? How does respiratory acidosis impact this planning?

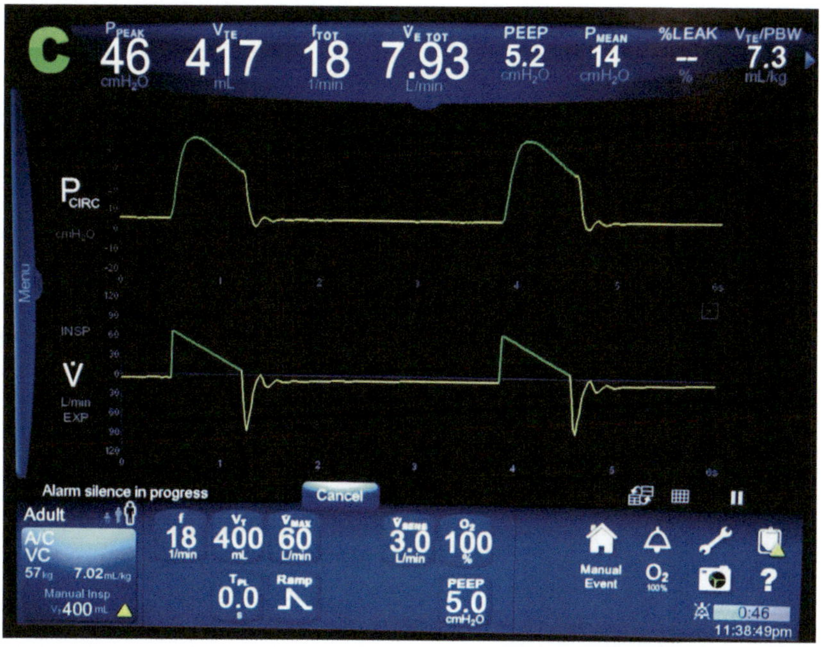

Fig. 19.4 Ventilator screen for Case 2

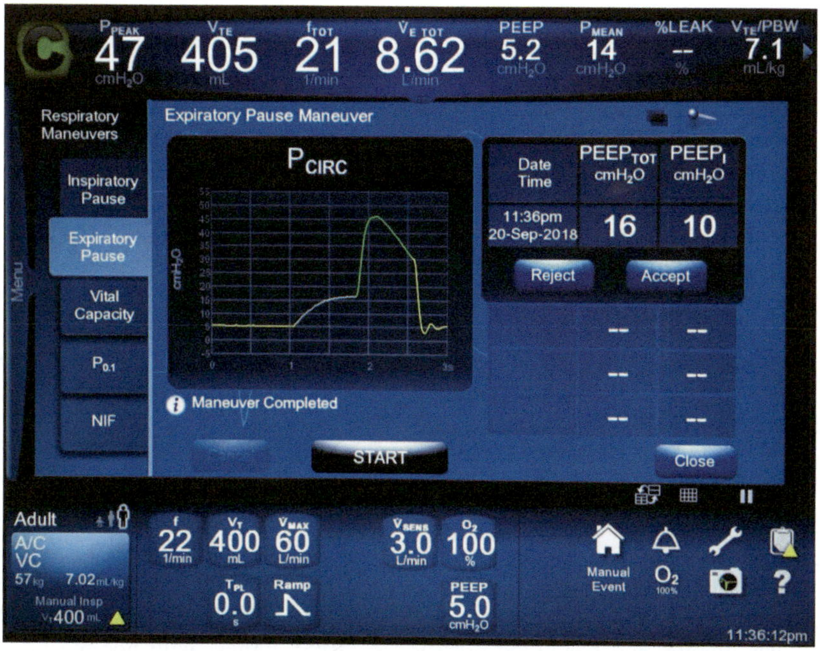

Fig. 19.5 Ventilator screen for Case 2

Case 2 Answers

1. The indications for intubation in asthma are hypoxemia and respiratory fatigue. The threshold to intubate is high, due to the risks of worsening air-trapping with mechanical ventilation. The air-trapping can lead to increased intrathoracic pressure, reducing venous return. This can result in life-threatening hemodynamic collapse.
2. This is assist control, volume control ventilation. Recall that assist control can be set to deliver a given volume (volume control) or a given pressure for a designated time (pressure control).
3. The tidal volume is 400 mL with a set rate of 18 breaths a minute. The set parameters are at the bottom of the screen, and the patient's response is at the top. This patient is not overbreathing, as the patient is receiving 18 breaths per minute. The exhaled tidal volume is 417 mL, very similar to the set value. Small differences (400–417) can be expected and are not abnormal.
4. After the increase in the respiratory rate, the autoPEEP, or intrinsic PEEP, is now 10–11 cmH_2O. The patient has a set PEEP of 5 cmH_2O, and the total PEEP is shown as 16 cmH_2O. AutoPEEP is additional intrathoracic pressure, and it can continue to increase. This likely developed due to a rapid respiratory rate and insufficient time to exhale. Increasing the respiratory rate in asthma (and often in COPD) can paradoxically lead to worse ventilation due to air-trapping. Permissive hypercapnia, or allowing a pH down to 7.15, is more appropriate. Ironically, slowing the rate will often allow for more complete exhalation and improved ventilation. Additionally, the increased intrathoracic pressure can result in hemodynamic collapse.
5. The team should disconnect the patient from the ventilator and gently exert pressure on her chest wall to assist with exhalation. They then should reconnect the ventilator but reduce the respiratory rate significantly, possibly to 10–12 breaths a minute.
6. In general, think "low." Lower tidal volumes (~6 mL/kg PBW) mean less volume to exhale. A low respiratory rate (8–12 breaths per minute) allows time to exhale. Low PEEP (~ 5 cmH_2O) reduces atelectasis while not inhibiting expiratory flow. As above, respiratory acidosis is tolerable in the short term while stabilizing a patient on the ventilator and allowing bronchodilators to work. Allowing time for exhalation is key to improving ventilation.

Case 3

A 58-year-old woman with a long history of smoking, possible COPD, and obesity presented to the hospital 2 days ago with pneumonia. Her hypoxemic respiratory failure required intubation and mechanical ventilation. Her chest X-ray is shown as Fig. 19.6. She is 5 feet, 5 inches tall, and she weighs 120 kg. Her heart rate is 115 beats per minute, and her blood pressure is 110/55 mmHg with norepinephrine

Fig. 19.6 Chest X-ray for Case 3

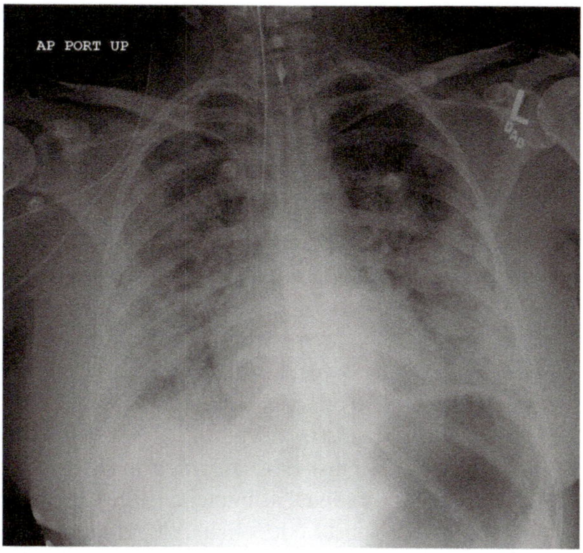

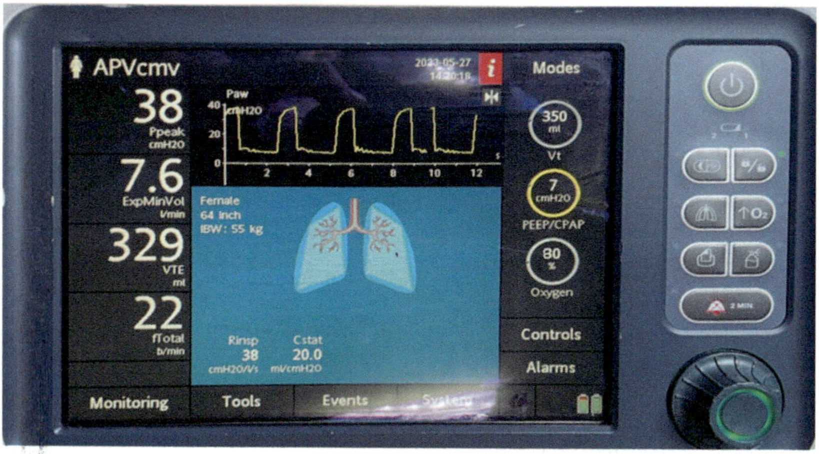

Fig. 19.7 Ventilator screen for Case 3

running at 10 μg/min. She is well-sedated on the ventilator, as shown in Fig. 19.7, and she is not overbreathing.

1. What is her tidal volume? What is your assessment of this value? Is it appropriate?
2. How does one define ARDS?
3. What is her PEEP? What is the PIP? What is her minute ventilation?
4. Does she have a compliance problem, a resistance problem, or both? What might contribute to each?

5. Her most recent ABG is 7.24/60/85 on 80% FiO_2. What is her PaO_2/FiO_2 ratio?
6. What are the options for managing her ventilator?
7. What additional options are available for improving her oxygenation?

Case 3 Answers

1. The patient's tidal volume is set at 350 mL. Using the ARDSnet table, this is roughly 6 mL per kilogram of predicted body weight. This is a perfectly appropriate starting tidal volume for most patients. In this scenario, however, the patient has very poor compliance, and her pressures seem high. The first step is to set a low tidal volume, but then, one must check to verify that the plateau pressure is less than 30 cmH_2O.
2. Acute respiratory distress syndrome (ARDS) is defined by four major criteria. First, the patient must have an acute insult causing respiratory failure within 7 days. Next, the patient has bilateral patchy infiltrates by chest radiography. The PaO_2/FiO_2 ratio must be less than 300 while on a positive pressure of at least 5 cmH_2O. Lastly, the condition cannot be explained fully by cardiogenic pulmonary edema.
3. Her PEEP is 7 cmH_2O and PIP 38 cmH_2O, and her minute ventilation is 7.6 L/min.
4. This ventilator provides the resistance and the compliance values. Her resistance is 38, which is extremely high. Additionally, her compliance is only 20, which is quite low. In this scenario, the patient has COPD, which likely contributes to a resistance issue, and she has ARDS, contributing to a compliance issue.
5. The ratio is 85/0.8 (for the 80% FiO_2). This leads to a ratio of 102.3 for borderline moderate to severe ARDS picture.
6. The first step is to bring down the patient's pressure if possible. She is receiving 6 mL per kg of predicted body weight, and this can be dropped to 5 or even 4. Her minute ventilation is only 7.6 L per minute, so her respiratory rate will need to be increased to compensate for the loss of tidal volume. The patient may respond to an increase in PEEP, possibly with a gentle recruitment maneuver, to improve her compliance and oxygenation.
7. If the patient does not respond to these maneuvers, she would be considered for proning as her PaO/FiO_2 ratio is less than 150. Additionally, while the inhaled pulmonary vasodilators epoprostenol and nitric oxide have not been proven to improve overall outcomes, they can be a bridge for transport and improve oxygenation. Lastly, if the patient continues not to improve, she should be evaluated by an ECMO team for VV ECMO. However, her prior history of COPD may preclude her from ECMO consideration, depending upon the severity and her overall prognosis.

Case 4

A 25-year-old man presents after multiple stab wounds, including one to the left chest. He is awake, alert, and to be transported to a trauma center. His initial chest X-ray did not show any acute pathology, but shortly before the arrival of the transport team, he develops shortness of breath and hypoxemia with an SpO_2 of 87% on room air. His repeat chest X-ray is shown in Fig. 19.8.

1. What is the cause of the patient's respiratory distress? What is the treatment?
2. What would be the risk of intubation before addressing the underlying issue?

   The patient has a chest tube placed but has continued instability. He becomes more confused and combative, with tachycardia at 125 beats per minute and hypotension with a blood pressure of 92/48 mmHg. After receiving blood, the patient remains altered and unstable, and the decision is made to intubate the patient for transport.
3. With presumed hemorrhage, what are the risks of intubation now?
4. How would you set the patient's ventilator? What additional data would you like to know?

   Figure 19.9 shows the ventilator screen.
5. What is the TV? What is minute ventilation? What is the PIP?
6. If this patient developed an undrained hemothorax, what changes would you expect to see on the ventilator?

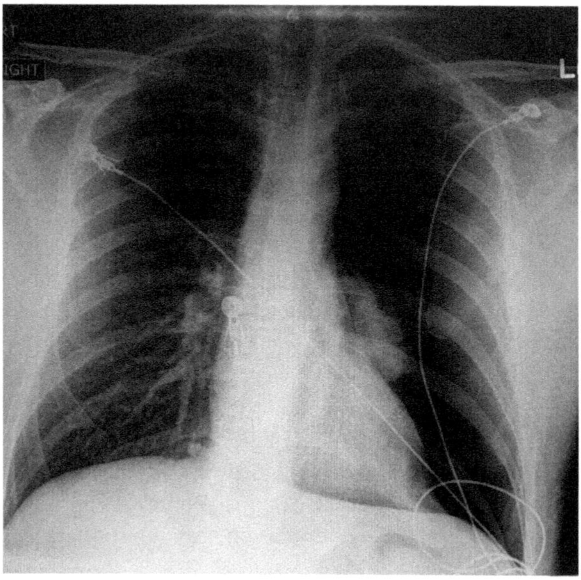

Fig. 19.8 Chest X-ray for Case 4

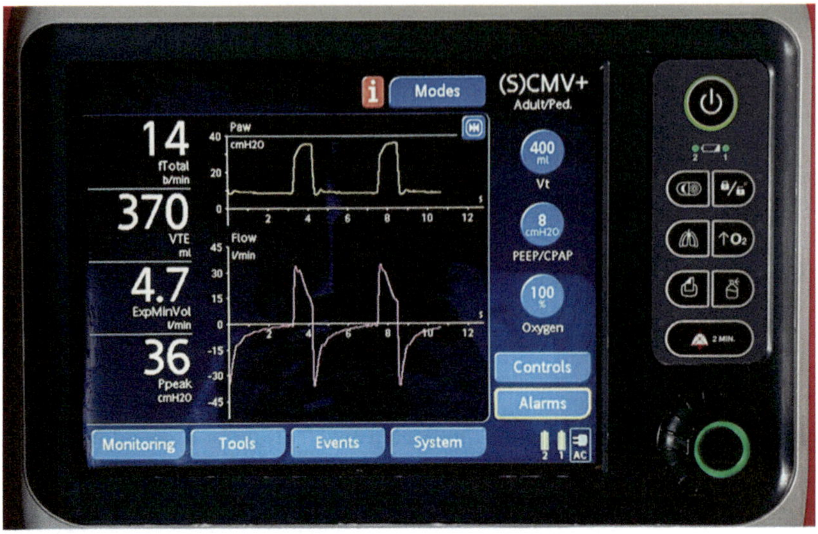

Fig. 19.9 Ventilator screen for Case 4

Case 4 Answers

1. This patient has a left-sided pneumothorax. If the patient is with clinicians who are qualified to place a chest tube, this is the appropriate treatment. If not, the patient should undergo a finger or needle thoracostomy and close monitoring until they arrive at a medical center where a chest tube can be placed.
2. If this patient were intubated and placed on positive pressure ventilation before the pneumothorax was addressed, the patient would be at risk of developing tension or worsening tension physiology. The application of positive pressure could increase the size of the pneumothorax and compress the mediastinum, resulting in hemodynamic collapse. Similarly, if this patient were taken to an elevated altitude without addressing the pneumothorax, the pneumothorax could also increase with gas expansion also leading to tension physiology.
3. With multi-trauma, the most common cause of preventable death is hemorrhage. Therefore, hemorrhage must always be on the differential for trauma patients. If this patient had a hemorrhage, intubation could worsen the hemodynamic status by increasing intrathoracic pressure and decreasing venous return in a system that is already volume-depleted.
4. This patient should be placed on lung protective ventilation with 6 mL/kg of predicted body weight. Trauma patients are at risk for the development of ARDS, and lung protective ventilation is an appropriate way to reduce this risk.

5. The tidal volume is 360 mL, the minute ventilation is 4.7 L/min, and the PIP is 36 cmH_2O.
6. In an undrained hemothorax, one would expect a decrease in compliance, resulting in an increase in the peak inspiratory pressure (PIP) and the plateau pressure (Pplat). With this patient being on a low tidal volume of 360 mL but with a high PIP of 36 cmH_2O, there should be concern for persistent pneumothorax or possibly hemothorax.

Case 5

The team is called to transport a 2-h-old girl, born at 29 3/7 weeks, weighing 1185 g. She was born to a 34-year-old G5, P4 mother. The mother presented overnight for premature rupture of membranes, and she underwent a STAT C-section with no delayed cord clamping. The neonate required positive pressure ventilation in the delivery room and had one failed intubation attempt. She was placed on CPAP and moved from the delivery room to the special care nursery, where she was then intubated on the second attempt.

1. What is a key intervention in a premature neonate who did not receive steroids while in utero, who undergoes an immediate intubation for respiratory distress?

   Surfactant was administered for RDS appearance on CXR, and an umbilical vein catheter was placed for hypotension. The patient had mean arterial pressures of 10–15 mmHg, with SBPs <20 mmHg.
2. What is on the differential diagnosis for this patient's hypotension?
3. What would be the next appropriate steps in management of this case?

   The patient does not have any evidence of a pneumothorax. Due to the hypotension, the patient received two normal saline boluses 10 mL/kg and started on dopamine from 5 to 7.5 μg/kg/min—now being transferred for neonatal intensive care which is not locally available.

   The team arrives in the Special Care Nursery to find a 2-h-old baby. Her fontanelle is soft and flat. She is intubated with a 3.0-mm tube, taped at 7.5 cm, and the ETT is confirmed with $ETCO_2$ monitoring. Her lung sounds are present bilaterally. Her ventilator screen is shown in Fig. 19.10.
4. What is the mode? What is the rate? Is this an appropriate rate for this child?
5. What is the FiO_2? Why is this level chosen?
6. What would be indications for high frequency oscillation ventilation?
7. Figure 19.11 shows the patient's venous blood gas. Does this indicate a need to increase the FiO_2?

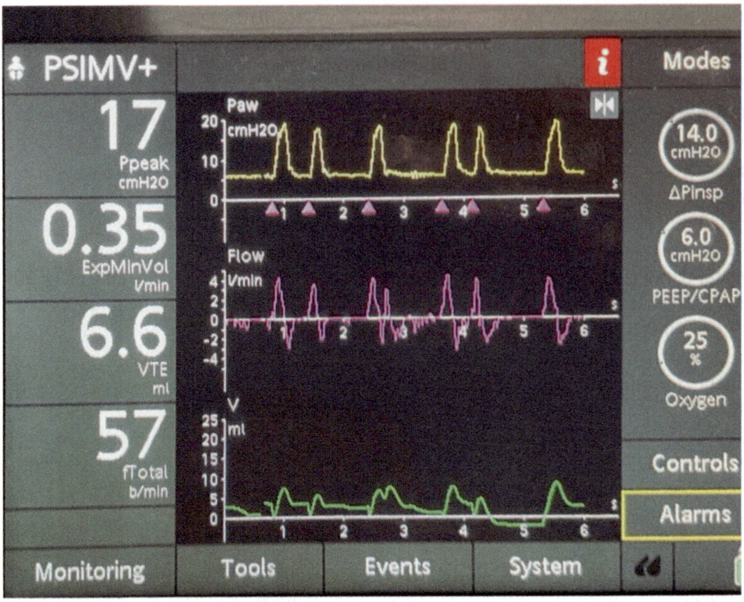

Fig. 19.10 Ventilator screen for Case 5

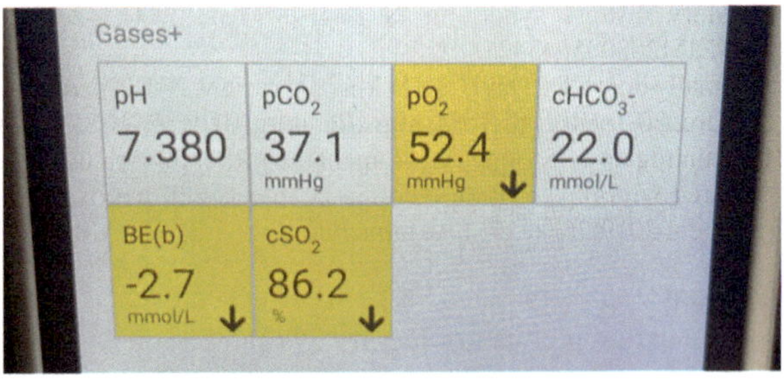

Fig. 19.11 Lab values for Case 5

Case 5 Answers

1. This patient is premature, and her mother presented with premature rupture of membranes. A C-section was apparently performed rapidly, and there was no time to administer steroids. As such, surfactant should be given after intubation to reduce the compliance.
2. The differential for this sick neonate is very similar to other patients—with sepsis and pneumothorax after ventilation being high on the list. She may also have a congenital disorder. While often diagnosed in utero, this unfortunately is not universal.
3. The patient should undergo transillumination of the chest to look for a pneumothorax. If there is no evidence of a pneumothorax, with the premature rupture of membranes, sepsis must be very high on the list. The patient should receive fluid

boluses at 10 cc/kg, up to 30 cc/kg, and then be started on dopamine for blood pressure support. The hemodynamic and ventilator support cannot be viewed in isolation, as the effects of one will impact the other.

4. This is synchronized intermittent mandatory ventilation, with pressure supported breaths between. It is set as pressure-targeted SIMV, for 14/6 of PEEP. The total rate is 57, which is a little high. However, considering that the neonate is likely septic, this elevated rate makes intuitive sense.
5. The FiO_2 is 25%. Although the baby needed intubation for respiratory support with surfactant administration and positive pressure, the oxygen requirements are not that high. The lowest effective FiO_2 should be used to reduce the risk of retinopathy of prematurity.
6. HFOV is most beneficial in patients with air leaks, lung hypoplasia, and pulmonary hypertension.
7. This gas is venous, likely taken from the umbilical vein catheter. A pO_2 on a venous gas is not a reliable marker of oxygenation and cannot be used to titrate FiO_2. The pH and pCO_2 on this gas are reassuring, however.

Further Reading

Acute Respiratory Distress Syndrome Network, Brower RG, Matthay MA, et al. Ventilation with lower tidal volumes as compared with traditional tidal volumes for acute lung injury and the acute respiratory distress syndrome. N Engl J Med. 2000;342(18):1301–8. https://doi.org/10.1056/NEJM200005043421801.

Ahmed SM, Athar M. Mechanical ventilation in patients with chronic obstructive pulmonary disease and bronchial asthma. Indian J Anaesth. 2015;59(9):589. https://doi.org/10.4103/0019-5049.165856.

Amato MBP, Meade MO, Slutsky AS, et al. Driving pressure and survival in the acute respiratory distress syndrome. N Engl J Med. 2015;372(8):747–55. https://doi.org/10.1056/NEJMsa1410639.

Askie LM, Darlow BA, Finer N, Schmidt B, Stenson B, Tarnow-Mordi W, Davis PG, Carlo WA, Brocklehurst P, Davies LC, Das A, Rich W, Gantz MG, Roberts RS, Whyte RK, Costantini L, Poets C, Asztalos E, Battin M, Halliday HL, Marlow N, Tin W, King A, Juszczak E, Morley CJ, Doyle LW, Gebski V, Hunter KE, Simes RJ, Neonatal Oxygenation Prospective Meta-analysis (NeOProM) Collaboration. Association between oxygen saturation targeting and death or disability in extremely preterm infants in the neonatal oxygenation prospective meta-analysis collaboration. JAMA. 2018;319(21):2190–201.

Barrocas M, Nuchprayoon CV, Claudio M, King FW, Danon J, Sharp JT. Gas exchange abnormalities in diffuse lung disease. Am Rev Respir Dis. 1971;104(1):72–87.

Brennan G, Colontuono J, Carlos C. Neonatal respiratory support on transport. Neoreviews. 2019;20(4):e202–12.

Combes A, Hajage D, Capellier G, et al. Extracorporeal Membrane Oxygenation for Severe Acute Respiratory Distress Syndrome. N Engl J Med. 2018;378(21):1965–75. https://doi.org/10.1056/nejmoa1800385.

Davis DP, Meade W, Sise MJ, Kennedy F, Simon F, Tominaga G, Steele J, Coimbra R. Both hypoxemia and extreme hyperoxemia may be detrimental in patients with severe traumatic brain injury. J Neurotrauma. 2009;26(12):2217–23.

de Moya M, Brasel KJ, Brown CVR, et al. Evaluation and management of traumatic pneumothorax: a Western Trauma Association critical decisions algorithm. J Trauma Acute Care Surg. 2022;92(1):103–7.

Donn SM, Mammel MC, van Kaam AHLC. Manual of neonatal respiratory care. Cham: Springer; 2022.

Duke HN, Killick EM. Pulmonary vasoconstriction to anoxia: its site of action. J Physiol. 1952;117(4):78P–9P.

Fan E, Del Sorbo L, Goligher EC, et al. An official American Thoracic Society/European Society of intensive care medicine/society of critical care medicine clinical practice guideline: mechanical ventilation in adult patients with acute respiratory distress syndrome. Am J Respir Crit Care Med. 2017;195(9):1253–63. https://doi.org/10.1164/rccm.201703-0548ST.

Gold MI, Helrich M. Pulmonary compliance during anesthesia. Anesthesiology. 1965;26:281–8.

Grieco DL, Chen L, Brochard L. Transpulmonary pressure: importance and limits. Ann Transl Med. 2017;5(14):285. https://doi.org/10.21037/ATM.2017.07.22.

Guérin C, Reignier J, Richard JC, et al. Prone positioning in severe acute respiratory distress syndrome. N Engl J Med. 2013;368(23):2159–68. https://doi.org/10.1056/nejmoa1214103.

Hatzfeld C, Wiener F, Briscoe WA. Effects of uneven ventilation-diffusion ratios on pulmonary diffusing capacity in disease. J Appl Physiol. 1967;23(1):1–10.

Laher AE, Buchanan SK. Mechanically ventilating the severe asthmatic. J Intensive Care Med. 2018;33(9):491–501. https://doi.org/10.1177/0885066617740079.

Levy BD, Kitch B, Fanta CH. Medical and ventilatory management of status asthmaticus. Intensive Care Med. 1998;24(2):105–17. https://doi.org/10.1007/S001340050530.

McFadden ER. Acute severe asthma. Am J Respir Crit Care Med. 2003;168(7):740–59. https://doi.org/10.1164/RCCM.200208-902SO.

Menk M, Estenssoro E, Sahetya SK, et al. Current and evolving standards of care for patients with ARDS. Intensive Care Med. 2020;46(12):2157–67. https://doi.org/10.1007/s00134-020-06299-6.

Mercat A, Richard JCM, Vielle B, et al. Positive end-expiratory pressure setting in adults with acute lung injury and acute respiratory distress syndrome: a randomized controlled trial. JAMA. 2008;299(6):646–55. https://doi.org/10.1001/jama.299.6.646.

Meyer K, Fernandes CJ, Schwartz HP. AAP Section on transport medicine. Neonatal content. Field guide for air and ground transport of neonatal and pediatric patients. 2018.

Mosier JM, Hypes C, Joshi R, Whitmore S, Parthasarathy S, Cairns CB. Ventilator strategies and rescue therapies for management of acute respiratory failure in the emergency department. Ann Emerg Med. 2015;66(5):529–41. https://doi.org/10.1016/J.ANNEMERGMED.2015.04.030.

National Heart, Lung and BIPCTN, Moss M, Huang DT, et al. Early neuromuscular blockade in the acute respiratory distress Syndrome. N Engl J Med. 2019;380(21):1997–2008. https://doi.org/10.1056/NEJMoa1901686.

Pai MP, Paloucek FP. The origin of the "ideal" body weight equations. Ann Pharmacother. 2000;34(9):1066–9. https://doi.org/10.1345/aph.19381.

Papazian L, Forel JM, Gacouin A, et al. Neuromuscular blockers in early acute respiratory distress syndrome. N Engl J Med. 2010;363(12):1107–16. https://doi.org/10.1056/NEJMoa1005372.

Papazian L, Aubron C, Brochard L, et al. Formal guidelines: management of acute respiratory distress syndrome. Ann Intensive Care. 2019;9(1):69. https://doi.org/10.1186/s13613-019-0540-9.

Peek GJ, Mugford M, Tiruvoipati R, et al. Efficacy and economic assessment of conventional ventilatory support versus extracorporeal membrane oxygenation for severe adult respiratory failure (CESAR): a multicentre randomised controlled trial. Lancet. 2009;374(9698):1351–63. https://doi.org/10.1016/S0140-6736(09)61069-2.

Pepe PE, Marini JJ. Occult positive end-expiratory pressure in mechanically ventilated patients with airflow obstruction: the auto-PEEP effect. Am Rev Respir Dis. 1982;126(1):166–70.

Petrucci N, De Feo C. Lung protective ventilation strategy for the acute respiratory distress syndrome. Cochrane Database Syst Rev. 2013;2013(2):CD003844. https://doi.org/10.1002/14651858.CD003844.pub4.

Ranieri VM, Rubenfeld GD, Thompson BT, et al. Acute respiratory distress syndrome: the Berlin definition. JAMA. 2012;307(23):2526–33. https://doi.org/10.1001/jama.2012.5669.

Sahetya SK, Goligher EC, Brower RG. Setting positive end-expiratory pressure in acute respiratory distress syndrome. Am J Respir Crit Care Med. 2017;195(11):1429–38. https://doi.org/10.1164/rccm.201610-2035CI.

Seethala RR, Frakes MA, Cocchi MN, et al. Feasibility and safety of prone position transport for severe hypoxemic respiratory failure due to coronavirus disease 2019. Crit Care Explor. 2020;2(12):e0293. https://doi.org/10.1097/cce.0000000000000293.

Silversides JA, Fitzgerald E, Manickavasagam US, et al. Deresuscitation of patients with iatrogenic fluid overload is associated with reduced mortality in critical illness. Crit Care Med. 2018;46(10):1600–7. https://doi.org/10.1097/CCM.0000000000003276.

Simon B, Ebert J, Bokhari F, Capella J, Emhoff T, Hayward T 3rd, Rodriguez A, Smith L. Management of pulmonary contusion and flail chest: an Eastern Association for the surgery of trauma practice management guideline. Eastern Association for the Surgery of Trauma. J Trauma Acute Care Surg. 2012;73:S351.

Slutsky AS, Ranieri VM. Ventilator-induced lung injury. N Engl J Med. 2013;369(22):2126–36. https://doi.org/10.1056/NEJMra1208707.

Spaite DW, Hu C, Bobrow BJ, Chikani V, Barnhart B, Gaither JB, Denninghoff KR, Adelson PD, Keim SM, Viscusi C, Mullins T, Sherrill D. The effect of combined out-of-hospital hypotension and hypoxia on mortality in major traumatic brain injury. Ann Emerg Med. 2017;69:62–72.

Talmor D, Sarge T, Malhotra A, et al. Mechanical ventilation guided by esophageal pressure in acute lung injury. N Engl J Med. 2008;359(20):2095–104. https://doi.org/10.1056/NEJMoa0708638.

Tomashefski JF. Pulmonary pathology of the adult respiratory distress syndrome. Clin Chest Med. 1990;11(4):593–619.

Tonetti T, Vasques F, Rapetti F, et al. Driving pressure and mechanical power: new targets for VILI prevention. Ann Transl Med. 2017;5(14):286. https://doi.org/10.21037/ATM.2017.07.08.

Ward NS, Dushay KM. Clinical concise review: Mechanical ventilation of patients with chronic obstructive pulmonary disease. Crit Care Med. 2008;36(5):1614–9. https://doi.org/10.1097/CCM.0B013E318170F0F3.

Watson WE. Some observations on dynamic lung compliance during intermittent positive pressure respiration. Br J Anaesth. 1962;34:153–7.

Conclusions and Key Concepts 20

Susan R. Wilcox

In summary, mechanical ventilation management is vital for critical care transport. As a reminder, the goals of this text are as follows

Familiarize Clinicians with Common Terms in Mechanical Ventilation

- Many terms are used interchangeably in mechanical ventilation, leading to confusion. Select appropriate terms and use them consistently.
- Key concepts include tidal volume, respiratory rate, minute ventilation, PEEP, resistance, compliance, peak inspiratory pressure, plateau pressure, autoPEEP, and derecruitment. Understanding the meaning of each term is crucial to understanding mechanical ventilation.
- Common modes of invasive mechanical ventilation are assist-control (including volume control and pressure control, as well as pressure-regulated volume control), synchronized intermittent mandatory ventilation, pressure support, and airway pressure release ventilation.

Review the Fundamental Principles of Pulmonary and Transport Physiology Relevant to Mechanical Ventilation

- There are two types of V/Q mismatch: Shunt is perfusion without ventilation, and dead space is ventilation without perfusion. The body tries to optimize V/Q matching by hypoxemic vasoconstriction. Shunt is a major cause of hypoxemia in transport.

S. R. Wilcox (✉)
Boston MedFlight, Bedford, MA, USA
e-mail: susan.r.wilcox@lahey.org

© The Author(s), under exclusive license to Springer Nature Switzerland AG 2024

S. R. Wilcox et al. (eds.), *Mechanical Ventilation in Critical Care Transport*,
https://doi.org/10.1007/978-3-031-66782-4_20

- Patients tend to derecruit after intubation and while lying supine. This is why PEEP is critical to maintaining oxygenation.
- Resistance involves flow, and compliance is the distensibility of the entire system. The peak inspiratory pressure includes both resistance and compliance; however, plateau pressure only involves compliance.
- Patients with respiratory failure tend to become unstable in transport. There are several mechanisms by which this occurs. Movement alone can result in V/Q mismatch, as can positioning requirements in transport.
- In flight, the reduced barometric pressure can expand air pockets, such as untreated pneumothoraces and bowel gas (Boyle's law). These should usually be decompressed before transport.
- Dalton's law states that as altitude increases, atmospheric pressure decreases, resulting in a decrease of the partial pressure of oxygen (PaO_2). Most people are not affected by this at typical rotor wing altitudes, but it may become relevant in patients with preexisting severe hypoxemia. Teams should be able to provide sufficient supplemental oxygen.

Discuss the Principles of Selecting Ventilator Settings

- Ventilator screens may provide a lot of data, but in general on most ventilators, the settings selected by the clinician, or control variables, appear along the bottom or the right side, and the patient's response, or the dependent variables, appears along the top. These can be shown as numerical values, as scalars (or waveforms), or as loops.
- Tidal volume should be selected for approximately 6 mL/kg of predicted body weight based on height and sex. The respiratory rate should be selected to target a reasonable minute ventilation, considering the patient's acid-base status. This will be 100–120 mL/kg PBW in someone with normal pH.
- PEEP should be set at a minimum of 5 cmH_2O in general and titrated higher as needed to correct for hypoxemia and derecruitment. The goal is to optimize compliance and oxygenation while not increasing the Pplat over 30 cmH_2O. The ideal PEEP will minimize both atelectasis and overdistention in the majority of the lungs.
- Once the ventilator settings are selected, the patient must be continuously reassessed. Settings such as those titrated based on blood gas and pulse oximetry must be monitored, and peak inspiratory pressures and plateau pressures must be monitored to reduce harm. End-tidal CO_2 ($EtCO_2$) is useful for trends but may not accurately reflect $PaCO_2$, particularly for patients in shock.

Develop Strategies for Transporting Ventilated Patients with ARDS and Severe Hypoxemic Respiratory Failure

- ARDS: The most important concept in the management of ARDS patients is low tidal volume ventilation while targeting a plateau pressure < 30 cmH_2O.
- These patients might also require high levels of PEEP for improved oxygenation. They may develop severe hypoxemia, even after intubation, requiring recruitment maneuvers to assist with oxygenation and neuromuscular blockade for ventilator synchrony.
- Additional techniques can be considered, including proning, the use of inhaled pulmonary vasodilators, and even ECMO.

Develop Strategies for Managing Asthma and COPD

- Asthma: These patients are at high risk of breath stacking, leading to autoPEEP. They should be ventilated with similarly low tidal volumes, a low respiratory rate, and low I:E ratios. They must be monitored for air trapping, and autoPEEP checked with an expiratory hold.
- COPD: COPD patients often respond well to BiPAP. If they require intubation, they should be treated very similarly to asthmatic patients. One difference is that patients with COPD may require higher levels of PEEP to match autoPEEP from collapsible distal airways.

Transport Patients with Neurologic Injury and Trauma

Neurologic injury: These patients are at risk for secondary injury during and after intubation from hypoxemia as well as hypocapnia. Therefore, efforts should be made not to hyperventilate these patients but instead to target normoxia and eucapnia.

Assess and Respond to Emergencies During Mechanical Ventilation

- Ventilator alarms should never be ignored and must always be investigated.
- The differential diagnosis for ventilator alarms is DOPES: Displacement, Obstruction, Pneumothorax, Equipment Failure, and Stacked Breathing.
- The mnemonic for action is DOTTS: Disconnect, Oxygen (bagging), Tube Position, Tweak the Vent, Sonography.

Further Reading

Acute Respiratory Distress Syndrome Network, Brower RG, Matthay MA, et al. Ventilation with lower tidal volumes as compared with traditional tidal volumes for acute lung injury and the acute respiratory distress syndrome. N Engl J Med. 2000;342(18):1301–8. https://doi.org/10.1056/NEJM200005043421801.

Ahmed SM, Athar M. Mechanical ventilation in patients with chronic obstructive pulmonary disease and bronchial asthma. Indian J Anaesth. 2015;59(9):589. https://doi.org/10.4103/0019-5049.165856.

Amato MBP, Meade MO, Slutsky AS, et al. Driving pressure and survival in the acute respiratory distress syndrome. N Engl J Med. 2015;372(8):747–55. https://doi.org/10.1056/NEJMsa1410639.

Askie LM, Darlow BA, Finer N, Schmidt B, Stenson B, Tarnow-Mordi W, Davis PG, Carlo WA, Brocklehurst P, Davies LC, Das A, Rich W, Gantz MG, Roberts RS, Whyte RK, Costantini L, Poets C, Asztalos E, Battin M, Halliday HL, Marlow N, Tin W, King A, Juszczak E, Morley CJ, Doyle LW, Gebski V, Hunter KE, Simes RJ, Neonatal Oxygenation Prospective Meta-analysis (NeOProM) Collaboration. Association between oxygen saturation targeting and death or disability in extremely preterm infants in the neonatal oxygenation prospective meta-analysis collaboration. JAMA. 2018;319(21):2190–201.

Barrocas M, Nuchprayoon CV, Claudio M, King FW, Danon J, Sharp JT. Gas exchange abnormalities in diffuse lung disease. Am Rev. Respir Dis. 1971;104(1):72–87.

Brennan G, Colontuono J, Carlos C. Neonatal respiratory support on transport. NeoReviews. 2019;20(4):e202–12.

Combes A, Hajage D, Capellier G, et al. Extracorporeal membrane oxygenation for severe acute respiratory distress syndrome. N Engl J Med. 2018;378(21):1965–75. https://doi.org/10.1056/nejmoa1800385.

Davis DP, Meade W, Sise MJ, Kennedy F, Simon F, Tominaga G, Steele J, Coimbra R. Both hypoxemia and extreme hyperoxemia may be detrimental in patients with severe traumatic brain injury. J Neurotrauma. 2009;26(12):2217–23.

de Moya M, Brasel KJ, Brown CVR, et al. Evaluation and management of traumatic pneumothorax: a Western trauma association critical decisions algorithm. J Trauma Acute Care Surg. 2022;92(1):103–7.

Donn SM, Mammel MC, van Kaam AHLC. Manual of neonatal respiratory care. Cham: Springer; 2022.

Duke HN, Killick EM. Pulmonary vasoconstriction to anoxia: its site of action. J Physiol. 1952;117(4):78P–9P.

Fan E, Del Sorbo L, Goligher EC, et al. An official American Thoracic Society/European society of intensive care medicine/society of critical care medicine clinical practice guideline: mechanical ventilation in adult patients with acute respiratory distress syndrome. Am J Respir Crit Care Med. 2017;195(9):1253–63. https://doi.org/10.1164/rccm.201703-0548ST.

Gold MI, Helrich M. Pulmonary compliance during anesthesia. Anesthesiology. 1965;26:281–8.

Grieco DL, Chen L, Brochard L. Transpulmonary pressure: importance and limits. Ann Transl Med. 2017;5(14):285. https://doi.org/10.21037/ATM.2017.07.22.

Guérin C, Reignier J, Richard JC, et al. Prone positioning in severe acute respiratory distress syndrome. N Engl J Med. 2013;368(23):2159–68. https://doi.org/10.1056/nejmoa1214103.

Hatzfeld C, Wiener F, Briscoe WA. Effects of uneven ventilation-diffusion ratios on pulmonary diffusing capacity in disease. J Appl Physiol. 1967;23(1):1–10.

Laher AE, Buchanan SK. Mechanically ventilating the severe asthmatic. J Intensive Care Med. 2018;33(9):491–501. https://doi.org/10.1177/0885066617740079.

Levy BD, Kitch B, Fanta CH. Medical and ventilatory management of status asthmaticus. Intensive Care Med. 1998;24(2):105–17. https://doi.org/10.1007/S001340050530.

McFadden ER. Acute severe asthma. Am J Respir Crit Care Med. 2003;168(7):740–59. https://doi.org/10.1164/RCCM.200208-902SO.

Menk M, Estenssoro E, Sahetya SK, et al. Current and evolving standards of care for patients with ARDS. Intensive Care Med. 2020;46(12):2157–67. https://doi.org/10.1007/s00134-020-06299-6.

Mercat A, Richard JCM, Vielle B, et al. Positive end-expiratory pressure setting in adults with acute lung injury and acute respiratory distress syndrome: a randomized controlled trial. JAMA. 2008;299(6):646–55. https://doi.org/10.1001/jama.299.6.646.

Meyer K, Fernandes CJ, Schwartz HP. AAP section on transport medicine. Neonatal content. Field guide for air and ground transport of neonatal and pediatric patients. 2018.

Mosier JM, Hypes C, Joshi R, Whitmore S, Parthasarathy S, Cairns CB. Ventilator strategies and rescue therapies for management of acute respiratory failure in the emergency department. Ann Emerg Med. 2015;66(5):529–41. https://doi.org/10.1016/J.ANNEMERGMED.2015.04.030.

National Heart, Lung and BIPCTN, Moss M, Huang DT, et al. Early neuromuscular blockade in the acute respiratory distress syndrome. N Engl J Med. 2019;380(21):1997–2008. https://doi.org/10.1056/NEJMoa1901686.

Pai MP, Paloucek FP. The origin of the "ideal" body weight equations. Ann Pharmacother. 2000;34(9):1066–9. https://doi.org/10.1345/aph.19381.

Papazian L, Forel JM, Gacouin A, et al. Neuromuscular blockers in early acute respiratory distress syndrome. N Engl J Med. 2010;363(12):1107–16. https://doi.org/10.1056/NEJMoa1005372.

Papazian L, Aubron C, Brochard L, et al. Formal guidelines: management of acute respiratory distress syndrome. Ann Intensive Care. 2019;9(1):69. https://doi.org/10.1186/s13613-019-0540-9.

Peek GJ, Mugford M, Tiruvoipati R, et al. Efficacy and economic assessment of conventional ventilatory support versus extracorporeal membrane oxygenation for severe adult respiratory failure (CESAR): a multicentre randomised controlled trial. Lancet. 2009;374(9698):1351–63. https://doi.org/10.1016/S0140-6736(09)61069-2.

Pepe PE, Marini JJ. Occult positive end-expiratory pressure in mechanically ventilated patients with airflow obstruction: the auto-PEEP effect. Am Rev. Respir Dis. 1982;126(1):166–70.

Petrucci N, De Feo C. Lung protective ventilation strategy for the acute respiratory distress syndrome. Cochrane Database Syst Rev. 2013;2013(2):CD003844. https://doi.org/10.1002/14651858.CD003844.pub4.

Ranieri VM, Rubenfeld GD, Thompson BT, et al. Acute respiratory distress syndrome: the Berlin definition. JAMA. 2012;307(23):2526–33. https://doi.org/10.1001/jama.2012.5669.

Sahetya SK, Goligher EC, Brower RG. Setting positive end-expiratory pressure in acute respiratory distress syndrome. Am J Respir Crit Care Med. 2017;195(11):1429–38. https://doi.org/10.1164/rccm.201610-2035CI.

Seethala RR, Frakes MA, Cocchi MN, et al. Feasibility and safety of prone position transport for severe hypoxemic respiratory failure due to coronavirus disease 2019. Crit Care Explor. 2020;2(12):e0293. https://doi.org/10.1097/cce.0000000000000293.

Silversides JA, Fitzgerald E, Manickavasagam US, et al. Deresuscitation of patients with iatrogenic fluid overload is associated with reduced mortality in critical illness. Crit Care Med. 2018;46(10):1600–7. https://doi.org/10.1097/CCM.0000000000003276.

Simon B, Ebert J, Bokhari F, Capella J, Emhoff T, Hayward T 3rd, Rodriguez A, Smith L. Management of pulmonary contusion and flail chest: an eastern Association for the Surgery of trauma practice management guideline. Eastern Association for the Surgery of Trauma. J Trauma Acute Care Surg. 2012;73:S351.

Slutsky AS, Ranieri VM. Ventilator-induced lung injury. N Engl J Med. 2013;369(22):2126–36. https://doi.org/10.1056/NEJMra1208707.

Spaite DW, Hu C, Bobrow BJ, Chikani V, Barnhart B, Gaither JB, Denninghoff KR, Adelson PD, Keim SM, Viscusi C, Mullins T, Sherrill D. The effect of combined out-of-hospital hypotension and hypoxia on mortality in major traumatic brain injury. Ann Emerg Med. 2017;53:443.

Talmor D, Sarge T, Malhotra A, et al. Mechanical ventilation guided by esophageal pressure in acute lung injury. N Engl J Med. 2008;359(20):2095–104. https://doi.org/10.1056/NEJMoa0708638.

Tomashefski JF. Pulmonary pathology of the adult respiratory distress syndrome. Clin Chest Med. 1990;11(4):593–619.

Tonetti T, Vasques F, Rapetti F, et al. Driving pressure and mechanical power: new targets for VILI prevention. Ann Transl Med. 2017;5(14):286. https://doi.org/10.21037/ATM.2017.07.08.

Ward NS, Dushay KM. Clinical concise review: mechanical ventilation of patients with chronic obstructive pulmonary disease. Crit Care Med. 2008;36(5):1614–9. https://doi.org/10.1097/CCM.0B013E318170F0F3.

Watson WE. Some observations on dynamic lung compliance during intermittent positive pressure respiration. Br J Anaesth. 1962;34:153–7.

Index

© The Editor(s) (if applicable) and The Author(s), under exclusive license to Springer Nature Switzerland AG 2024
S. R. Wilcox et al. (eds.), *Mechanical Ventilation in Critical Care Transport*, https://doi.org/10.1007/978-3-031-66782-4

R

S

T

V

GPSR Compliance

The European Union's (EU) General Product Safety Regulation (GPSR) is a set of rules that requires consumer products to be safe and our obligations to ensure this.

If you have any concerns about our products, you can contact us on ProductSafety@springernature.com

In case Publisher is established outside the EU, the EU authorized representative is:

Springer Nature Customer Service Center GmbH
Europaplatz 3
69115 Heidelberg, Germany

Batch number: 10412353

Printed by Printforce, the Netherlands